Lecture Notes in Computer Science 2526

Edited by G. Goos, J. Hartmanis, and J. van Leeuwen

T0232290

Springer

Berlin
Heidelberg
New York
Barcelona
Hong Kong
London
Milan
Paris
Tokyo

Alfredo Colosimo   Alessandro Giuliani
Paolo Sirabella (Eds.)

Medical
Data Analysis

Third International Symposium, ISMDA 2002
Rome, Italy, October 10-11, 2002
Proceedings

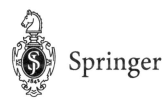 Springer

Series Editors

Gerhard Goos, Karlsruhe University, Germany
Juris Hartmanis, Cornell University, NY, USA
Jan van Leeuwen, Utrecht University, The Netherlands

Volume Editors

Alfredo Colosimo
Paolo Sirabella
Dept. of Human Physiology and Pharmacology
University of Rome La Sapienza
P. le A. Moro, 5, 00185 Rome, Italy
E-mail:
a.colosimo@caspur.it
paolo.sirabella@uniroma1.it

Alessandro Giuliani
TCE Laboratory, Istituto Superiore di Sanità
V. le Regina Elena, 299, 00161 Rome, Italy
E-mail: alessandro.giuliani@iss.it

Cataloging-in-Publication Data applied for

Bibliograhpic information published by Die Deutsche Bibliothek
Die Deutsche Bibliothek lists this publication in the Deutsche Nationalbibliografie;
detailed bibliographic data is available in the Internet at http://dnb.ddb.de

CR Subject Classification (1998): I.2, H.2.8, H.3, G.3, I.5.1, I.4, J.3, F.1

ISSN 0302-9743
ISBN 3-540-00044-5 Springer-Verlag Berlin Heidelberg New York

Springer-Verlag Berlin Heidelberg New York
a member of BertelsmannSpringer Science+Business Media GmbH

http://www.springer.de

© Springer-Verlag Berlin Heidelberg 2002
Printed in Germany

Typesetting: Camera-ready by author, data conversion by Boller Mediendesign
Printed on acid-free paper   SPIN: 10873138   06/3142   5 4 3 2 1 0

Preface

The International Symposium on Medical Data Analysis is an important periodical opportunity to exchange ideas and first-hand experiences with groups interested in the medical applications of innovative hardware and software tools.

The massive information available through continuous improvements in the various modeling approaches to Medical Data Analysis is reflected in the results, dealing with quite different topics, presented during the Third Edition of the Symposium (ISMDA 2002). They have been grouped into the following four categories: (1) Data Mining and Decision Support Systems; (2) Medical Informatics and Modeling; (3) Time-Series Analysis; and (4) Medical Imaging.

In setting up the symposium program we tried to avoid, even with the shortage of time, parallel sessions. Thus, all participants had the chance to catch all the oral presentations, and we hope that this third proceedings volume will extend this chance also to non-participants. As for the previous volumes, it contains extensive up-to-date chapters on Medical Data Analysis, packed with ideas, suggestions, and solutions to many problems typical of this field.

An appealing feature of ISMDA is the informal character coupled to a careful selection and reviewing procedure for the submitted contributions, which guaranteed a high-quality standard within a relaxing and friendly environment. In this connection, it is not only fair but also a great pleasure for us to thank the many people involved in the set-up of ISMDA 2002, from the authors to the organizing committee to the international panel of reviewers, all of them provided an invaluable contribution to the success of the symposium.

September 2002

Alfredo Colosimo
Alessandro Giuliani
Paolo Sirabella

Organization

The ISMDA 2002 symposium was organized by the CISB, the Interdepartmental Research Centre for Models and Information Analysis in Biomedical Systems, University of Rome, La Sapienza, Italy.

Scientific Committee

A. Babic   Linköping University, Sweden
R. Brause   J.W. Goethe University, Germany
A. Colosimo   University of Roma, La Sapienza, Italy
S. Cerutti   Polytechnic School, Milano, Italy
N. Ezquerra   Georgia Tech., USA
A. Giuliani   Nat. Inst. of Health, Italy
J. Hasenkam   Aarhus University, Denmark
H.G. Holzütter   Humboldt University of Berlin, Germany
E. Keravnou   University of Cyprus, Cyprus
P. Larranaga   University of the Basque Country, Spain
N. Lavrac   J. Stefan Institute, Slovenia
R. Lefering   University of Köln, Germany
A. Macerata   Institute of Clinical Physiology, Italy
V. Maojo   Polytechnical University of Madrid, Spain
E. Neugebauer   University of Köln, Germany
C. Ohmann   University of Heine, Germany
L. Ohno-Machado   Harvard Univ., USA
A. Pazos   University of A. Coruña, Spain
L. Pecen   Acad. of Sciences of the Czech Republic, Czech Republic
W. Sauerbrei   University of Freiburg, Germany
B. Sierra   University of the Basque Country, Spain
B. Silverman   University of Pennsylvania, USA
J. Sima   Acad. of Sciences of the Czech Republic, Czech Republic
P. Sirabella   University of Rome, La Sapienza, Italy
H. Sitter   University of Marburg, Germany
J.P. Zbilut   Rush University, Chicago, USA
B. Zupan   University of Ljubljana, Slovenia

Table of Contents

Data Mining and Decision Support Systems

Medical Informatics and Modeling

Time-Series Analysis

Medical Imaging

Knowledge Discovery Using Medical Data Mining

Fernando Alonso[1], África López-Illescas[2], Loïc Martínez[1], Cesar Montes[3],
Juan P. Valente[1]

[1]Dept. Languages & Systems, [3]Dept. Artificial Intelligence, Univ. Politécnica de Madrid
Campus de Montegancedo s/n, Boadilla, Madrid
{falonso, loic, cmontes, jpvalente}@fi.upm.es
[2]High Performance Centre, Madrid, Spanish Council for Sports
africa.lopez@csd.mec.es

Abstract: In this paper we describe the process of discovering underlying knowledge in a set of isokinetic tests (continuous time series) using data mining techniques. The methods used are based on the discovery of sequential patterns in time series and the search for similarities and differences among exercises. They were applied to the processed information in order to **characterise injuries** and **discover reference models** specific to populations. The discovered knowledge was evaluated against the expertise of a physician specialised in isokinetic techniques and applied in the I4 project (Intelligent Interpretation of Isokinetic Information)[1].

1   Introduction

This paper describes the knowledge discovery component of a medical diagnosis system in the field of physiotherapy and, more specifically, in muscle function assessment. The system processes data received from an isokinetic machine, using expert systems and data mining techniques.

An isokinetic machine (Figure 1a) can be described as a piece of apparatus on which patients perform strength exercises. This machine has the peculiarity of limiting the range of movement and the intensity of effort at a constant velocity (which explains the term isokinetic).

Data concerning the strength employed by the patient throughout the exercise are recorded and stored in the machine so that physicians can collect and visually analyse the results using specialised computer software. Figure 1b shows the result of one exercise as a strength curve.

The information produced by isokinetic machines has a wide range of applications not only in physiotherapy, but also in orthopedics and other medical specialities. The principle is quite simple: the device moves at a constant speed through all the possible angles, at the same time as the patient pushes it using the part of the body that is under examination (in our case, knee flexions and extensions). If everything is in order the

---

[1] The I4 has been developed in conjunction with the Spanish National Centre for Sports Research and Sciences and the School of Physiotherapy of the Spanish National Organisation for the Blind. It has been funded by the Spanish Ministry of Science and Technology.

A. Colosimo et al. (Eds.): ISMDA 2002, LNCS 2526, pp. 1-12, 2002.

increase or decrease in the strength exerted by the person at each consecutive angle should be somehow continuous. On the other hand, large fluctuations in the strength exerted are indicative of some kind of injury or disease.

All the tests are performed following strict protocols that ensure that enough and the right data are collected for each patient. In our case, the exercises are performed following a protocol specified by the expert, which consists of a total number of six exercises: three different speeds (60°/s, 180°/s and 300°/s) performed with each leg.

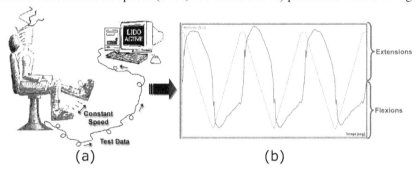

Fig. 1. Diagram of isokinetics machine (1a) and the resultant data (1b).

The potential of isokinetic machines for therapists is indiscutable. However, inexperience and the shortage of references is still the major problem. It is very difficult for a novice to understand and analyse the results, and even experts experience problems as they have no reference models to aid decision making on a particular test. Moreover, different kinds of populations (grouped by age, injury, profession, etc.) behave differently, which leads to different categories of curves.

Data mining techniques on time series were required to analyse isokinetic exercises in order to discover new and useful information for later use in a range of applications. Patterns discovered in isokinetic exercises performed by injured patients are very useful, especially for monitoring injuries, detecting potential injuries early or discovering fraudulent sicknesses. These patterns are also useful for the creation of reference models for population groups that share some characteristics.

2   Overview of the System

I4 is a rather large system that combines knowledge discovery in databases (KDD) and knowledge-based systems (KBS) approaches to help physicians to understand and use isokinetic data. This is a really difficult task as a lot of experience is needed to understand the meaning of the data provided by isokinetic machines, and it can be very hard, even for experts, to build reference models or patterns to help them make the right decisions.

Figure 2 shows the functional structure of the I4 system. First, data collected from the isokinetic machine are pre-processed to build a clean and normalised database. The pre-processing tasks are performed in two steps. I4 first decodes, transforms, formats and stores the original input in a standard format and corrects any inaccurate or incomplete data. The data cleaning and pre-processing module then automatically corrects and removes any inconsistencies between the isokinetic tests, using intelligent expert knowledge-based techniques.

Once the data have been prepared they can be either directly displayed or automatically processed using any of the two main analysis components. The first one is a KBS used to analyse individual exercises [1]. The KBS provides an expert knowledge-based analysis of the isokinetic curves related to both their numerical parameters and their morphology. It lightens the workload of experienced physicians in isokinetics and provides support for non-specialists.

The second one is a KDD system, which is the focus of this paper. It is composed of two main modules. The input of the characterise injuries module is exercises representative of any particular injury, which it uses to discover sequential models in time series in order to detect patterns repeated across more than one isokinetic exercise. These patterns can then be used to classify the injuries that occur. The goal of the create reference models module is to build reference curves for a given patient population. To do this, it identifies and discards any atypical curves and then searches for similarities within the curves of the patient population. For this purpose, the fast Fourier transform is used to convert the curves into a frequency domain, thus leading to a more efficient search for similarities [2] [3].

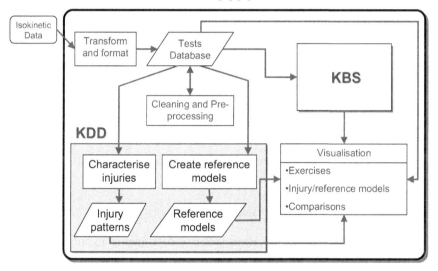

Fig. 2. Overview of the I4 system

Both modules, and the innovative approaches that they employ will be described in detail in the following.

3   Knowledge Discovery

Data was collected and prepared before executing the data mining process. These tasks are described very briefly below. The pre-processing phase is described in detail in [1].

- **Collecting initial data**. This collection of data was composed of close to 1580 isokinetic tests. The tests include the personal particulars of the patient and six isokinetic exercises. Each exercise is a series of 350 to 600 triplets of real numbers (strength, angle, time). All this amounted to just over 103 Mbytes of information.
- **Preparing the data**. This task involved the following actions: data analysis and decoding, creation of the I4 database, expert cleaning of data (removal of incorrect tests, elimination of incorrect extensions and flexions) and expert pre-processing. Expert knowledge had to be used to automatically remove the irregularities in the strength curves caused by isokinetic machine inertia and retain deviations that were due to the strength exerted by patients. Figure 3 shows a diagram of the data preparation tasks

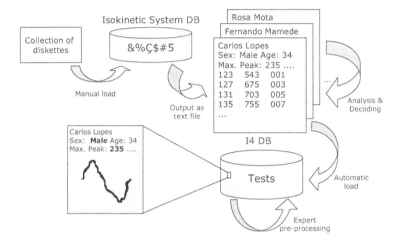

Fig. 3. Data pre-processing tasks

3.1   Detecting Injury Patterns in Isokinetic Exercises

One of the most important potential applications of data mining algorithms for this sort of time series is to detect any parts of the graph that are representative of an irregularity. As far as isokinetic exercises are concerned, the presence of this sort of alterations could correspond to some kind of injury, and correct identification of the alteration could be an aid for detecting the injury in time. So, the identification of patterns, that is, portions of data that are repeated in more than one graph, is of vital importance for being able to establish criteria by means of which to classify the exercises and, therefore, patients.

Method for Discovering Characteristic Injury Patterns
The process of developing a DM method to identify patterns that potentially characterise some sort of injury was divided into two phases:

1. Develop an algorithm that detects similar patterns in exercises.
2. Use the algorithm developed in point 1 to detect any patterns that appear in exercises done by patients with injuries and do not appear in exercises completed by healthy individuals.

The problem defined in phase 1) of the method of injury identification is set out as follows:

- Given:
  - A collection S of time series, composed of sequences of values (usually real numbers) of variable length, where the length of the longest is *max-length.*
  - The value (supplied by the user) of minimum confidence *min-conf* (number of series in which a pattern appears divided by the total number of series).
  - The maximum distance between patterns to be considered similar (*max-dist*).

- Find:
  - All frequent patterns present in S, that is, identical or similar sequences that appear in S with a confidence greater or equal to *min-conf.*

A pattern search tree was built in order to speed up the pattern-searching algorithm. Each depth level of this tree coincides with the length of each pattern, that is, a branch of depth 2 corresponds to a given pattern of length 2. In identical pattern-searching algorithms [4], it suffices to store the pattern and a counter of appearances in each node. When dealing with continuous data, however, similar patterns have to be considered and, therefore, the list of series in which the pattern appears (SA) and the list of series in which a similar pattern appears (SSA) have to be stored (Figure 4). This is because pattern similarity does not have the property of transitivity (we can have p1 similar to p2, p2 similar to p3 and p1 not similar to p3).

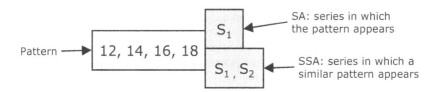

Fig. 4. Format of a similar pattern search tree node.

Major changes had to be made to state-of-the-art algorithms in order to consider similar patterns, as these algorithms either search for identical patterns in the series or consider only patterns of a given length. In the identical pattern-searching algorithms, each pattern matches a branch of the tree. In the similar pattern-searching algorithm in question, however, a pattern can match several branches, depending on the specified distance *max-dist*. For example, taking *max-dist* = 1, the patterns {12, 14, 16, 18} and {12, 14, 16, 19} are considered similar, and this must be taken into account when calculating the frequency of the two patterns.

First, the algorithm builds candidate patterns that appear in the time series in the same manner as an identical pattern-searching algorithm would do. To calculate pattern frequency, however, it is not enough just to store the number of times the pattern appears in the series. It is important to find out in which series the pattern appears in order to be able to analyse its similarity with other patterns. The identifiers of the series in which each candidate pattern appears are stored in the SA field of each node. Then the algorithm has to run through the candidate patterns to modify the SSA set, taking into account the appearances attributed to similar candidate patterns. For each candidate pattern, all the candidate patterns of the same length in the tree that are at a lesser distance than threshold *max-dist* are considered similar patterns, and the respective SSA sets are updated with the series from the SA set of the other similar node. Obviously, identical patterns are also considered to be similar, which means that the SSA sets of a node are initialised with the SA set of the node in question (SA ⊆ SSA).

Special care has to be taken in the pruning phase not to prune candidate patterns, which, although not themselves frequent, play a role in making another pattern frequent. If this sort of candidate patterns were pruned, the algorithm would not be complete, that is, would not find all the possible patterns. Only candidate patterns that are infrequent and whose minimum distance from the other patterns is further than the required distance will be pruned. Having completed the tree-pruning phase, the next level of the tree is generated using the longest patterns.

The algorithm steps are described in detail below.

Step 1.   Scan the time series database looking for sub-sequences of length i (starting with length 1) and enter the series in which each sub-sequence (candidate pattern) is detected into the respective SA set.

Step 2.   Calculate the distance between pairs of candidate patterns for all the candidate patterns of length i, provided the calculated distance is less than defined by the user (*max-dist*), and update the SSA sets of the nodes of the two candidate patterns by adding the series belonging to the SA set of the other pattern. That is, for two similar patterns p1 and p2, SSA(p1) = SSA(p1) ∪ SA(p2). The confidence of a candidate pattern is calculated with the SSA set.

Step 3.   Prune the search tree. To be pruned, a node must satisfy two conditions: a) the candidate pattern in the node must not be frequent, that is, its confidence must be less than specified (*min-conf*); b) the minimum distance of the candidate pattern in the node to the other patterns must be greater than the maximun similarity distance defined by the user (max-dist). This assures that infrequent candidate patterns that could be part of longer patterns (in future iterations of the algorithm) and could possibly raise the confidence of other patterns in the future are not pruned.

Step 4.   Return to Step 1 if not all the nodes of the branch of the tree have been pruned and candidate patterns of length $i + 1$ can be built.

This algorithm is able to search a large set of time series of non-homogeneous lengths, finding the patterns (time subsequences of undetermined length) that are repeated in any position of a significant number of series. Therefore, the algorithm will be useful for finding significant patterns that are likely to characterise a set of non-uniform time series, even though important characteristics of these patterns, like length or position within the time series, are unknown.

Example of Algorithm Application

Given the pattern series: $S_1 = \{1, 0, 1\}$, $S_2 = \{1, 1, 1\}$ and $S_3 = \{2, 2, 1\}$, with *max-length*=3, the algorithm will be applied with the parameters *min-conf*=0.75 and *max-dist*=1.

During the first algorithm iteration, three patterns of length 1 are found in the series. Pattern $\{0\}$ appears in S_1, pattern $\{1\}$ appears in S_1, S_2, S_3 and pattern $\{2\}$ appears in S_3. Pattern $\{0\}$ is similar to pattern $\{1\}$ (Euclidean distance = 1) and, therefore, the SSA for pattern $\{0\}$ includes the three series. The same applies to pattern $\{2\}$. Finally, pattern $\{1\}$ is similar to patterns $\{0\}$ and $\{2\}$, but these two patterns add no new information to the SSA of pattern $\{1\}$. In the pruning step, the confidence level of all three patterns in the SSA series is high (1.0), and all three patterns are kept for the next iteration.

In the second iteration, there are only five patterns of length 2 that appear in at least one of the series: $\{0,1\}$, $\{1,0\}$, $\{1,1\}$, $\{2,1\}$ and $\{2,2\}$. Pattern $\{0,1\}$ is only similar to pattern $\{1,1\}$, as is pattern $\{1,0\}$. Pattern $\{1,1\}$ is similar to $\{0,1\}$, $\{1,0\}$ and $\{2,1\}$. Pattern $\{2,1\}$ is similar to $\{1,1\}$ and $\{2,2\}$. Finally, pattern $\{2,2\}$ is only similar to $\{2,1\}$.

In the pruning step, only pattern $\{1,1\}$ has a high enough confidence level. However, patterns $\{0,1\}$, $\{1,0\}$ and $\{2,1\}$ are similar to pattern $\{1,1\}$ and are, therefore, also kept for the next iteration. The only pattern to be pruned in this iteration is $\{2,2\}$ (because it is not frequent and its minimum distance to the other patterns is greater than the maximun similarity distance *max-dist*).

In the third and last iteration, there are only two patterns of length 3 that appear in any of the series: $\{1,0,1\}$ in S_1 and $\{1,1,1\}$ in S_2. Both patterns are similar and their SSAs are updated. These patterns are pruned, because their confidence is low and there are no similar patterns with a high confidence level.

The algorithm ends here with only four possible patterns having a high enough confidence level: $\{0\}$, $\{1\}$, $\{2\}$ and $\{1,1\}$. Figure 5 summarises this example.

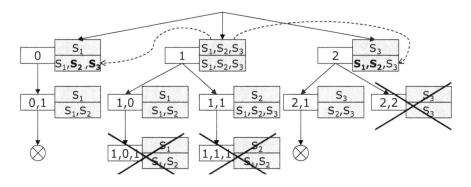

Fig. 5. Similar pattern search tree

Real Example

A real example of similar pattern-searching algorithm application to pattern detection in isokinetic exercises is shown below. In this case, we had a set of eight exercises completed by injured female patients (knee cartilage disease). This is a feasible number, because it is difficult to find more patients with the same sort of injury for evaluation in a given environment (in this case, Spanish top-competition athletes). The graphs of the exercises used are shown in Figure 6.

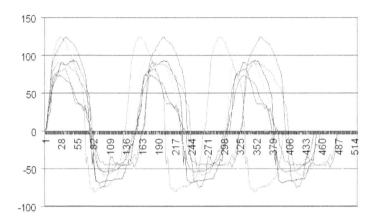

Fig. 6. Eight isokinetic exercises performed by injured patients (knee cartilage disease)

The problem is to detect patterns symptomatic of knee cartilage disease. Taking the exercises shown in Figure 6, the similar pattern-searching algorithm finds a number of patterns, the most promising of which is shown in Figure 7a. This pattern corresponds to the lower part of the curves, as shown in Figure 7b. Note that the discovered patterns do not necessarily appear at the same point in all series, which overcomes problems, such as a possible time deviations between different patients' series. We then tried to match this pattern against a set of healthy patients' exercises, and this pattern did not show up. After a positive expert evaluation, we will be able to use this pattern as a symptom of knee cartilage disease.

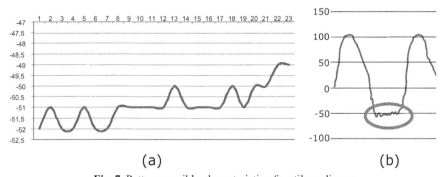

(a)   (b)

Fig. 7. Pattern possibly characteristic of cartilage disease

3.2   Creation of Reference Models for Population Groups

One of the most common tasks involved in the assessment of isokinetic exercises is to compare a patient's test against a reference model created beforehand. These models represent the average profile of a group of patients sharing common characteristics.

All the exercises done by individuals with the desired characteristics of weight, height, sport, sex, etc., must be selected to create a reference model for a particular population. However, there may be some heterogeneity even among patients of the same group. Some will have a series of particularities that make them significantly different from the others. Take a sport like American football, for instance, where players have very different physical characteristics. Here, it will make no sense to create a model for all the players, and individual models would have to be built for each subgroup of players with similar characteristics. Therefore, exercises have to be discriminated and the reference model has to be created only with exercises among which there is some uniformity.

It was the expert in isokinetics who used to be responsible for selecting the exercises that were to be part of the model. Discarding any exercises that differ considerably from the others is a job that is difficult to do manually. This meant that it was mostly not done. The idea we aim to implement is to automatically discard all the exercises that are different and create a model with the remainder.

Once the user has selected all the tests of the patient population to be modelled, the process for creating a new reference model is as follows (there is a preliminary pre-processing phase, also affecting the other system modules, which removes the irregularities in the graph caused by system inertia rather than the patient's strength; furthermore, any full extensions and flexions incorrectly performed by the patient are also removed):

1. Calculate the fast Fourier transform of the series (once the series has been pre-processed, only the first 256 values are used).
2. Class the first four coefficients of the Fourier transform of these exercises, using a clustering algorithm. These four coefficients are enough to represent the curve trends. Thus, the groups of similar exercises are clearly identified as they are grouped into different classes.
3. Normally, users mostly intend to create a reference model for a particular group, and there is clearly a majority group of similar exercises, which represents the standard profile that the user is looking for, and a disperse set of groups of one or two exercises. The former are used to create a reference model, in which all the common characteristics of the exercises are unified.

   The first step for creating the actual model is normalisation. This step levels out the size of the different isokinetics curves and adjusts the times when patients exert zero strength (switches from flexion to extension and vice versa), as these are singular points that should coincide in time. The second step is to calculate the mean value of the curves point to point. Finally, we apply the pattern discovery algorithm to the group of exercises and add every pattern found as an attribute of the model. This last step is taken because, when calculating the average curve, patterns may be smoothed if they appear at different moments in time in the exercises.

4. An isokinetic exercise for a patient, or a set of isokinetic exercises, will later be able to be compared with the models stored in the database. Thus, we will be able to determine the group to which patients belong or should belong and identify what sport they should go in for, what their weaknesses are with a view to improvement or how they are likely to progress in the future.

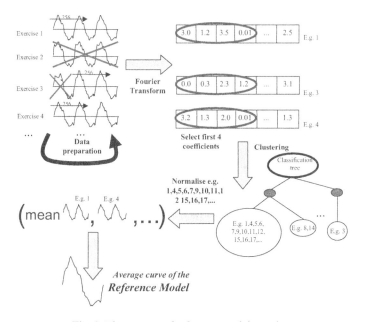

Fig. 8. The process of reference model creation

4   Evaluation and Conclusions

The discovered knowledge was difficult to evaluate because there was little sound background knowledge about most of the populations under study. Furthermore, even acknowledged experts experience great difficulty in assessing the quality of a model.

Therefore, the evaluation process focused on, first, verifying whether the output models where representative of the populations and to what extent and, second, validating their fitness for achieving the selected goals: pattern-based injury detection and model-based population characterisation

The sources of knowledge for both evaluations were confined to the experts, the cases database, the few existing models and everyday practice. So, the whole process had to be carefully planned as a long-term evaluation, based on a five-step procedure:

1. Subjective appraisal of the results by the experts.
2. Comparison of the results with previous known cases. These were very limited as the only available sources were the cases themselves and a few existing models.

3. Turing Test-based validation tests, in which the effectiveness of the discovered knowledge was compared against the expert. This task was planned to get a neat idea of the strength of the results when applied in everyday practice.
4. Continuous daily evaluation with real–life cases. This is a corrective stage and will continue throughout the research project life cycle.
5. Evaluation of satisfaction, whose goal is to gain an understanding of the feelings of practitioners when the results derived from DM are applied in everyday practice.

For a more thorough discussion of each of the evaluation tasks performed in I4, see [1]. Here, we will just outline the results obtained in step #3. The results are shown in Tables 1 and 2.

Table 1. Evaluation of injury detection.

Injury detection scenario			
	System	Expert	Novice
15 common injuries	15 OK	15 OK	Failed 2
5 uninjured	4 OK and 1 don't know	5 OK	3 OK (no mistakes)
5 rare injuries	Detected as rare cases (no mistakes)	2 mistakes and 1 don't know	3 don't knows

Table 2. Evaluation of reference models creation.

Reference models			
	System	Expert	Novice
30 members	4 mistakes	9 mistakes	21 mistakes
10 non- members	No mistakes	No mistakes	No mistakes
10 unclassified	No mistakes	2 mistakes	2 mistakes

We can conclude that the results obtained with the KDD modules surpass the expected results. Obviously, these results must be read carefully, as most of the mistakes made by practitioners can be put down to the fact that they were working without sound background knowledge of many diseases and had to deal with a huge amount of data for decision making. In this respect, I4 was at an advantage. Anyhow, the same practitioners have found I4 to be an extremely useful tool, and are currently using two versions of the system [5]. The first, called ES for Isokinetics Interpretation *(ISOCIN)*, was designed for use by visually impaired physicians, so all the information presented to the user is voice synthesised. This system can be used without a display. *ISOCIN* is currently being used by blind physicians at *Spanish Organisation for the Blind's School of Physiotherapy* to analyse injuries in any kind of patient and assess their evolution, adapting the physiotherapy administered and the rehabilitation process. The other application, an ES for Interpreting Isokinetics in Sport *(ISODEPOR)*, is being used at the National High Performance Centre to evaluate the muscle strength of Spanish top-competition athletes.

References

1. Alonso F, Valente J P, López-Chavarrías I, Montes C (2001a) Knowledge discovery in time series using expert knowledge. Medical Data Mining and Knowledge Discovery, Physica-Verlag, pp 455-496.
2. Agrawal R, Faloustsos C and Swami A (1993) Efficient similarity search in sequence databases, In: Proc. of Foundations of Data Organisations and Algorithms FODO.
3. Faloutsos C, Ranganathan M and Manolopoulos Y (1994) Fast subsequence matching in time series databases, In: Proc. of SIGMOD 94, Minneapolis, pp 419-429.
4. Han J, Dong G and Yin Y (1998) Efficient mining of partial periodic patterns in time series database, In: Proc. of Fourth International Conference on Knowledge Discovery and Data Mining, AAAI Press, Menlo Park, pp 214-218.
5. Alonso F, Valente J P, López-Illescas A, Martínez L, Montes C (2001b) Analysis of Strength Data Based on Expert Knowledge. LNCS 2199 Medical Data Analysis, Springer, pp 35-41.
6. Valente J P , López-Chavarrías I (2000) Discovering patterns in time series, In: Proc of 6th Intl. Conf. on Knowledge Discovery and Data Mining KDD, Boston, pp 497-505.

Analysis of Stationary Periods of Heart Rate via Symbolic Dynamics

Camillo Cammarota[1], Giuseppe Guarini[2], and Maria Ambrosini[2]

[1] Department of Mathematics
[2] 2nd Department of Cardiology
University of Rome 'La Sapienza', p.le A. Moro 2, 00185, Rome, Italy

Abstract. In recent literature the reduced heart rate variability has been recognized as an adverse sign in several heart diseases. In the present paper a new measure of variability based on the research of stationary periods of heart rate in symbolic dynamics is introduced. Stationary periods are defined in terms of accelerations and decelerations of the instantaneous rate in strips of four consecutive qualified beats. Using this definition we compare the amount of stationary periods of the electrocardiographyc sinusal R-R intervals both in clinically healthy and in transplanted subjects to the ones in atrial fibrillation. The R-R sequences are provided by the Holter ECG of 12 recipient subjects transplanted from at least 5 years, of 18 healthy subjects and 18 subjects presenting only atrial fibrillation. Despite the comparability of the mean heart rate of the three groups, the amount of stationary periods was found to be significantly larger in transplanted than in healthy. The amount of stationary periods in fibrillating subjects turns out to have an intermediate value; this value can be explained assuming that in the symbolic dynamics the R-R intervals appears to be a sequence of independent random variables. The larger amount of stationary periods in transplanted subjects can suggest a reduced or absent autonomic nervous regulation.

1 Introduction

The heart rate is characterized by more or less ample fluctuations due to different factors (e.g. prevalent sympathetic or vagal domain, catecholamines or acethilcolines hyperincretions, breathing activity, etc.). It is well known that the reduced heart rate variability in the cardiocirculatory insufficiency and in post-heart infarct clinical course is a warning sign. From some AA. a connection between sudden death and reduced variability has been demonstrated ([1]- [7]). Various quantitative definitions of variability can be given ([8]). The related notion of complexity has also been investigated as related to the aging ([9], [10]) The variability of heart beat is less known in the cardiac recipient. In literature the works about this problem are very rare and limited to the study of spectral analysis of some strips of the 24h Holter. Furthermore the results published are not univocal.

In the present paper we consider the heart variability as characterized by a variable amount of stationary or non-stationary periods. The definitions are

A. Colosimo et al. (Eds.): ISMDA 2002, LNCS 2526, pp. 13–19, 2002.

given in the context of the symbolic dynamics associated to the heartbeat sequence. In a previous paper we studied the amounts of stationary heart rate in normal subjects and cardiac recipients with an analytic method recently elaborated by us ([11]-[14]). In the present study we extend the analysis to a group of subjects with only atrial fibrillation.

2   Methods

We studied 12 recipient subjects that were transplanted at least 5 years before with ages between 25 and 45 years. All the patients, chosen from those followed by our laboratory, at the time of our research presented a very good post-operative course. Only a few presented in anamnesis a previous episode of allograft-reaction that had been promptly well remitted. At the time of our research the patients had an optimal cardiocirculatory performance. We have also studied 18 subjects with only atrial fibrillation. A control test was carried out on 18 normal subjects 27-45 years old chosen from medical and nursing staff from our cardiologyc department. In all the patients the 24h Holter of cardiac beats was divided into strips of four successive beats. Automatically all the strips of four beats which presented artifacts or ectopic atrial or ventricular beats were eliminated. The strips with these defects varied from case to case but were never more than 20% of the total Holter recording.

Our definition of stationary periods is based on the construction of a symbolic dynamics associated to the tachogram. If two consecutive R-R intervals are of increasing duration we associate to them a + mark and if they are of decreasing duration we associate a - mark. Notice that + mark means deceleration of the heart rate and a - mark means acceleration of the heart rate. In the present study for sake of simplicity we have chosen to eliminate the strips such that at least two consecutive intervals were of the same duration.

The remaining strips were subdivided into three groups.

The first group is formed by strips such that the sequence of the four beats presents exactly 3 accelerations or 3 decelerations (i.e. - - - or + + +). We call these strips of 'type zero' and the total frequency of occurrence is denoted p_0.

The second group is formed by strips in which the sequence of the four beats presents accelerations or decelerations for at least two consecutive beats (i.e. - - +, - + +, + - -, + + -). We call these strips of 'type one' and the total frequency of occurrence is denoted p_1.

The third group is formed by strips in which accelerations and decelerations are alternating (i.e. + - + and - + -). We call these strips of 'type two' and the total frequency of occurrence is denoted p_2.

We call 'stationary periods' the strips of the third group and the frequency p_2 is an indicator of the amount of stationary periods.

By definition one has

$$p_0 + p_1 + p_2 = 1$$

hence there are only two independent quantities.

We have considered a simple mathematical model based on a sequence, denoted $X_0, X_1, X_2, \ldots$ of independent random variables uniformly distributed on the interval $[0,1]$. In this model an exact evaluation of the frequencies of the occurrence of the three events above defined can be easily performed computing the corresponding probabilities. For instance one has

$$p_0 = \text{Prob}(+++) + \text{Prob}(---)$$

$$= \text{Prob}(X_0 < X_1 < X_2 < X_3) + \text{Prob}(X_0 > X_1 > X_2 > X_3)$$

The first summand is

$$\text{Prob}(X_0 < X_1 < X_2 < X_3) = \int_0^1 dx_0 \int_{x_0}^1 dx_1 \int_{x_1}^1 dx_2 \int_{x_2}^1 dx_3$$

$$= \int_0^1 dx_0 \int_{x_0}^1 dx_1 \int_{x_1}^1 dx_2 (1 - x_2)$$

$$= \int_0^1 dx_0 \int_{x_0}^1 dx_1 \left(\frac{1}{2} - x_1 + \frac{x_1^2}{2} \right)$$

$$= \int_0^1 dx_0 \left(\frac{1}{6} - \frac{1}{2}x_0 + \frac{1}{2}x_0^2 - \frac{1}{6}x_0^3 \right) = \frac{1}{24}$$

Carrying out similar calculations one gets for the frequencies the values

$$p_0 = \frac{1}{12}, \quad p_1 = \frac{1}{2}, \quad p_2 = \frac{5}{12}$$

The pseudo random sequence generated by the computer simulates this type of variables. A sequence of length comparable to the one of the tachogram has been analyzed with our counting algorithm and the frequencies were found very near to the theoretical ones. In order to compare these values with the ones from measurement we use the percent rounded values

$$p_0 \sim 8.3\% \quad p_1 \sim 50.0\% \quad p_2 \sim 41.7\%$$

3   Results

The results that we obtained with this methodology are reported in the following tables containing percent rounded values; N denotes normal, T transplant and F fibrillation. Here p_0, p_1, p_2 denote percentage and of course in each row one has $p_0 + p_1 + p_2 = 100$.

normal	p_0	p_1	p_2	fibrillation	p_0	p_1	p_2
$N1$	17	60	23	$F1$	8	50	42
$N2$	20	59	21	$F2$	10	52	38
$N3$	23	57	20	$F3$	9	51	40
$N4$	15	64	21	$F4$	9	52	39
$N5$	25	48	27	$F5$	9	51	40
$N6$	23	52	25	$F6$	8	49	43
$N7$	15	59	26	$F7$	8	49	43
$N8$	18	58	24	$F8$	9	51	40
$N9$	29	53	18	$F9$	11	52	37
$N10$	25	55	20	$F10$	8	51	41
$N11$	25	50	25	$F11$	9	49	42
$N12$	16	64	20	$F12$	10	51	39
$N13$	20	67	13	$F13$	9	49	42
$N14$	20	67	13	$F14$	10	52	38
$N15$	26	55	19	$F15$	9	51	40
$N16$	18	59	33	$F16$	10	51	39
$N17$	17	60	23	$F17$	9	52	39
$N18$	19	65	16	$F18$	9	51	40
average	20.6	58.4	21.0	average	9.1	50.8	40.1
st.dev.	4.2	5.6	4.1	st.dev.	0.8	1.1	1.7

transplant	p_0	p_1	p_2
$T1$	5	44	51
$T2$	4	44	52
$T3$	4	45	51
$T4$	4	46	50
$T5$	16	42	42
$T6$	11	44	45
$T7$	4	45	51
$T8$	2	36	62
$T9$	3	42	55
$T10$	5	45	50
$T11$	10	40	50
$T12$	4	41	55
average	6.0	42.8	51.2
st.dev.	4.1	2.8	5.0

4   Discussion

The most evident result is that the symbolic dynamics in atrial fibrillation is well described using as a model of the RR intervals a sequence of independent random variables. The physiological interpretation of this result is subjected to the following two cautions.

Firstly we have assumed that the distribution in our model is uniform in order to have a simpler evaluation of the frequencies. A more accurate computation should use the real distribution of the RR intervals, but its mathematical form is not known.

Secondly our results suggest that the symbolic dynamics of the fibrillation is near to be random and uncorrelated, but this cannot be said of the entire dynamic. The correlations that characterize the real dynamics could be partially explained using the presence of deterministic trends in the RR sequence. We remark that at least the linear trends are eliminated by our method, since the quantities estimated are defined only in terms of the differences.

The complex behavior of the heart rate dynamics in normal subjects depends on both the control of the autonomic nervous systems and the pacing action of the sino atrial node (autochthonous heart activity). In heart recipient subjects, the activity of the heart is expressed by normal sino-atrial rhythm which presents itself immediately after the transplant. Both autonomic and autochthonomic regulation of heart beats may be influenced by physical, chemical and hormonal stimuli. Both may support stationary and non-stationary rates even if on average in normal subjects appears evident from the results of our research that the non stationary rates are greater than in other groups. This is probably due to the autonomic nervous regulation that allows the immediate functional adaptation of heart rate.

In the transplanted patients the cardiac muscle is a denervated muscle even if some AA. have hypothesized a process of re-innervation after some years as time goes by ([15]-[19]). This is not our opinion because studying the phase space and spectral analysis of 24h Holter files in our transplanted patients, who were in periodic observation in the last 5 years in 2nd Cardiologyc Institute, we have never demonstrated a cardiac re-innervation [20].

It is therefore evident that the more frequent and longer periods of stationary state of heart beats in transplanted patients can be referred to a reduced or absent regulation of the autonomic nervous system.

In this way the observation in these patients of the higher incidence of stationary strips of pulse speed is indicative of a pendular rhythm. As it is known this rhythm is characteristic of premature newborns and babies in the first days of life. This phenomenon is commonly referred to as an incomplete development of the autonomic nervous system.

References

1. Kleiger R.E., Miller J.P., Bigger J.T., Moss A.J. and the Multicenter Post-Infarction Research Group, Decreased heart rate variability and its association with increased mortality after acute myocardial infarction, Am. J. Cardiol. 59:256-262
2. De Ferrari G.M., Vanoli E., Scwartz P.J., Cardiac vagal activity myocardial ischemia and sudden death. In Zipes D.P. Jalife J. eds. Cardiac Electrophysiology: From Cell to Bedside. Philadelphia, Pa: W.B. Saunders Co. 422-434 (1995)

3. Davidenko J.M., Pertsov A.V., Salomonsz R. Baxter W., Jalife J., Stationary and drifting spiral waves of excitation in isolated cardiac muscle Nature 23: 349-351(1992)

4. Copie X., Hnatkova K., Blankoff I., Staunton A., Camm A.J., Malik M., Risque de mortalite apres un infarctus du myocarde: apport de la frequence cardiaque, de sa variabilite, et de la fraction d'ejection ventriculaire gauche. Arch Mal Coeur Vaiss, 89 (7) 865-71 (1996)

5. Copie X., Le Heuzey J.Y., Iliou M.C., Pousset F., Lavergne T., Guize L., Evolution de la variabilite de la frequence cardiaque apres infarctus du myocarde. Apport du diagramme de Poincare. Arch Mal Coeur Vaiss 88 (11)1621-6 (1995)

6. Heart rate variability. Standards of Measurement , Physiological Interpretation , and Clinical Use . Task Force of the European Society of Cardiology and the North American Society of Pacing and Electrophysiology Circulation 93:1043-1065 (1996)

7. Copie X., Hnatkova K., Staunton A., Fei L., Camm A.J., Malik M., Predictive power of increased heart rate versus depressed left ventricular ejection fraction and heart rate variability for risk stratification after myocardial infarction. Results of a two-year follow-up study. J Am Coll Cardiol. 27 (2) 270-6 (1996)

8. Kurths,J., Voss, A., Saparin, P., Kleiner H. J., Wessel, N. Quantitative analysis of heart rate variability, Chaos 5, 88-94 (1995).

9. Giuliani,A., Colosimo, A. Complexity and aging as correlated with heartbeat dynamics, Proceedings of 'Complexity in the living: a modelistic approach' Rome, CISB (1998)

10. Colosimo, A., Giuliani, A., Mancini, A.M., Piccirillo, G., Marigliano, V., Estimating a cardiac age by means of heart rate variability, Am. J. Physiol., H1841-H1847 (1997).

11. Ambrosini M., Cammarota C., Guarini G., Heart rate stationarity in heart transplanted patients. Clin Ter 152 (6)363-366 (2001)

12. Cammarota C., Ambrosini M., Sette A., Di Luozzo M.,Nesta C., Rotunno R., Sellitti I., Sulla variabilit dell'attivit cinetica del cuore nei cardiotrapiantati Atti 102 Cong. Naz. Soc. Ital Med. Int. S 13 2001-11-04

13. Cammarota C., Ambrosini M., Sette A., Di Luozzo M., Nesta C., Rossi P., A new mathematical method for thr analysis of the presumed reinnervation of the transplanted heart. Atti VIII National Congress of the Italian Society of Cardiovascular research. Turin Italy 20-22 September 2001 Italian Heart J. Vol. 2 Suppl.

14. Ambrosini M., Rossi P., Sette A., Nesta C., Di Luozzo M., Cammarota C., The presumed reinnervation of the transplanted human heart: analysis with a new mathemetical method. Marilleva, Trento 2002

15. Meyer M;, Marconi C., Ferretti G., Fiocchi R, Cerretelli P, Skinner J.E., Heart rate variability in the human transplanted heart: nonlinear dynamics and QT vs RR-QT alterations during exercise suggest a return Integr Physiol Behav Sci 31(4):289-305 (1996)

16. Fallen E.L.,Kamath M.V., Ghista D.N., Fitchett D., Spectral Analysis of heart rate variability following human heart transplantation evidence for functional reinnervation J Auton. Nerv. Syst. 23:199-206 (1988)

17. Arrowood J.A. Goudreau E. Minisi A.J. Davis A.B. Mohanty P.K. Evidence against reinnervation of cardiac vagal afferents after human orthotopic cardiac transplantation Circulation 92:402-408 (1995)

18. Rowan R.A., Billingham M.E., Myocardial innervation in long-term heart transplant survivors: a quantitative ultrastructural survey J Heart Transplant 7:448-452 (1988)

19. Meyer M, Marconi C, Ferretti G, Fiocchi R, Cerretelli P, Skinner JE, Heart rate variability in the human transplanted heart: nonlinear dynamics and QT vs RR-QT alterations during exercise suggest a return of neurocardiac regulation in long-term recovery. Integr Physiol Behav Sci 31(4):289-305(1996)
20. Guarini G., Cammarota C., Fidente D., Marino O. andAmbrosini M. The auto-correlation of cardiac beat as a method of research of the heart's memory (First communication) Clin.Ter.149:215-217(1998)

Microcalcification Detection Using a Kernel Bayes Classifier

B. Caputo (*,+), E. La Torre (+), G.E. Gigante (+)

(*) Smith-Kettlewell Eye Research Institute 2318 Fillmore Street, San Francisco 94115 California, USA, caputo@ski.org
(+) University of Rome 'La Sapienza', CISB- Physics Department, Piazza A. Moro 3, 00161, Rome, Italy
fb.caputo, elatorre, g.giganteg@caspur.it

Abstract. Mammography associated with clinical breast examination is the only effective method for mass breast screening. Microcalcifications are one of the primary signs for early detection of breast cancer. In this paper we propose a new kernel method for classification of dificult to diagnose regions in mammographic images. It consists of a novel class of Markov Random Fields, using techniques developed within the context of statistical mechanics. This method is used for the classification of positive Region of Interest (ROI's) containing clustered microcalcifications and negative ROI's containing normal tissue. We benchmarked the new proposed method with a nearest neighbor classifier and with an artificial neural network, widely used in literature for computer-aided diagnosis. We obtained the best performance using the novel approach.

1 Introduction

The usage of machine learning algorithm for the development of computer assisted diagnosis system is a well developed area of research [11, 19]. The diagnostic process is a very complicated procedure, the outcome of which depends on numerous factors. Some of these factors relate to the procedure itself and others are associated with characteristics of the human visual system. In the situation in which all technical factors are at a high quality level, the human factor becomes more important. The perception of details and the recognition of the meaning of these details are the weakest links in the biomedical image interpretation process; perceptual and cognitive problems occur that will result in loss of information and a lower quality of the resulting diagnosis. Thus the importance of developing computer-assisted diagnosis systems which make use of knowledge developed within the machine learning community.

A challenging application problem is the detection of microcalcifications in X-ray mammograms. Screen-films mammography associated with clinical breast examination and breast self examination is widely recognized as the only effective imaging modality for early detection of breast cancer in women [16, 7]. However, the interpretation of X-ray mammograms is very difficult because of the small differences

A. Colosimo et al. (Eds.): ISMDA 2002, LNCS 2526, pp. 20-31, 2002.

in the image densities of various breast tissues, particularly for dense breast. The interpretation of mammograms by radiologists is performed by a visual examination of films for the presence of abnormalities that indicate cancerous changes. Computerized analysis might be of significant value to improve the true-positive rate of breast cancer detection. Among the early indicators of breast cancer, microcalcifications are one of the primary signs. They are tiny granule-like depositum of calcium, and the presence of clustered microcalcifications in X-ray mammograms is considered a basic marker for the early detection of breast cancer, especially for individual microcalcification with diameters up to about 0.7 *mm* and with an average diameter of 0.3 *mm* [16, 7]

Computerised image analysis methods have been used for the identification of circumscribed masses, classification of suspicious areas and classification of microcalcifications using conventional methods [10], [15] and using expert systems [10]. In the actual interpretation of mammographic microcalcifications, the gray-level values defining local structures in the microcalcification clusters play a significant role [7]. It has been demonstrated in clinical studies described in [7], that the grouping of microcalcification regions, in order to define the shape of the cluster, is highly dependent on the gray-level-based structure and texture of the image.

Texture information plays an important role in image analysis and understanding, with potential applications in remote sensing, quality control, and medical diagnosis. Texture is one of the important characteristics used in identifying an object or a region of interest (ROI) in an image [6]. A vast literature has addressed this topic in the last decades [10, 11, 6, 19, 15, 3]. Most of work has been devoted to the search of key textural features for the representation of significant information. The classification step is generally performed using Artificial Neural Networks (ANN)

In this paper we focus the attention on the choice of the classification algorithm rather than on the choice of the textural features. We propose to use Spin Glass - Markov Random Fields (SG-MRF, [4]) for microcalcification detection. SG-MRF is a fully connected MRF which integrates results of statistical physics of disordered systems [1] with Gibbs probability distributions via non linear kernel mapping [14]. SG-MRF have shown to be very effective for many visual applications such as appearance-based object recognition, texture classification and so forth [4]. Here we apply the very same strategy for microcalcification detection. We represent each Region Of Interest (ROI) using a shape histogram representation [13], then we model the SG-MRF on the histogram bins. This probabilistic model is used to classify ROI into positive ROIs containing microcalcifications and negative ROIs containing normal tissue. The classification step is performed using a Maximum A Posteriori (MAP) probability classifier. We compare SG-MRF's performance with that obtained using a Nearest Neighbor Classifier (NNC) and an ANN given by a three-layer perceptron, with backpropagation learning algorithm. In all the experiments we performed, SG-MRF obtained the best performances. To the best of our knowledge, these are the first experiments on microcalcification detection that show a better performance of a given method (in this case SG-MRF) with respect to a multi-layer perceptron classifier.

The paper is organized as follows: Section 2 describes the algorithm used for the feature extraction step. Section 3 reviews basic concepts of ANN, Section 4 reviews Bayes classifiers and Section 5 summarizes the SG-MRF model and how it can be employed for classification purposes in a MAP classifier. Section 6 presents experimental results; the paper concludes with a summary discussion.

2 Feature Extraction: Multidimensional Receptive Field Histograms

Multidimensional receptive Field Histograms (MFH) were proposed by Schiele [13] in order to extend the color histogram approach of Swain and Ballard [17]. The main idea is to calculate multidimensional histograms of the response of a vector of receptive fields. A MFH is determined once we chose the local property measurements (i.e., the receptive field functions), which determine the dimensions of the histogram, and the resolution of each axis. On the basis of the results reported in [4], we chose to use in this research work two local characteristics based on Gaussian derivatives:

$$D_x = -\frac{x}{\sigma^2} G(x, y), \ D_y = -\frac{x}{\sigma^2} G(x, y), \tag{1}$$

Where

$$G(x, y) = \exp\left(-\frac{x^2 + y^2}{2\sigma^2}\right) \tag{2}$$

is the Gaussian distribution. The parameter σ explicitly determines the scale of the filter, and it will be specified later.

3 Artificial Neural Networks

Also referred to as connectionist architectures, parallel distibuted processing, and neuromorphic systems, an artificial neural network (ANN) is an information-processing paradigm inspired by the way the densely interconnected, parallel structure of the mammalian brain processes information. Artificial neural networks are collections of mathematical models that emulate some of the observed properties of biological nervous systems and draw on the analogies of adaptive biological learning. The key element of the ANN paradigm is the novel structure of the information processing system. It is composed of a large number of highly interconnected processing elements that are analogous to neurons and are tied together with weighted connections that are analogous to synapses [8], [12], [2]. A weight w_{ij} (coupling strength) characterizes the interconnections between any two neurons i and j. The input to each neuron is a weighted sum of the outputs incoming from the connected neurons. Each neuron operates on the input signal using his activation function f and produces the output response. The typical activation functions are linear, threshold and sigmoid [12], [2].

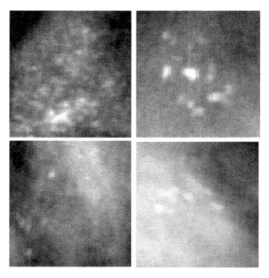

Fig. 1. Four examples of ROIs containing microcalcifications

Normally the neurons are organized in an architecture with input nodes, interfacing the neural network and the external world, output nodes, producing the network's responses, and hidden nodes, having the task of correlating and building up an "internal representation" of the analyzed problem. Network's capacity and performance depends on the number of neurons, on the activation functions used, and on the neurons' interconnections. Another important attribute of artificial neural networks is that they can efficiently learn nonlinear mappings through examples contained in a training set, and use the learned mapping for complex decision making [12], [2].

Although ANNs have been around since the late 1950's, it wasn't until the mid-1980's that algorithms became sophisticated enough for general applications. Today ANNs are being applied to an increasing number of real-world problems of considerable complexity. They are good pattern recognition engines and robust classifiers, with the ability to generalize in making decisions about imprecise input data. The advantage of ANN lies in their resilience against distortions in the input data and their capability of learning. They are often good at solving problems that are too complex for conventional technologies (e.g., problems that do not have an algorithmic solution or for which an algorithmic solution is too complex to be found) and are often well suited to problems that people are good at solving, but for which traditional methods are not.

4 Probabilistic Bayes Classifier

Let $\mathbf{x} \equiv [x_{ij}]$; $i = 1; \ldots N$; $j = 1; \ldots M$ be an $M \times N$ image. We will consider each image as a feature vector $x \in G \equiv \Re^m$; $m = MN$. Assume we have k different classes $\Omega_1, \Omega_2, \ldots, \Omega_k$, of visual objects, and that for each visual object is given a set of n_j data samples, $d_j = \{x_1^j, x_2^j, ..., x_{n_j}^j\}$, j = 1; . . . k. We will assign each visual object to a pattern class Ω_1, Ω_2,..., Ω_k,. The classification procedure will be a discrete mapping that assigns a test image to the pattern class it corresponds to.

The probabilistic approach to appearance-based visual object recognition considers the image views of a given visual object Ω_j as random vectors. Thus, given the set of data samples d_j and assuming they are a sufficient statistic for the pattern class Ω_j, the goal will be to estimate the probability distribution $P_{\Omega j}(x)$ that has generated them. Then, given a test image x, the decision will be made using a Maximum A Posteriori (MAP) classifier:

$$j^* = \underset{j}{\operatorname{argmax}}\, P_{\Omega_j}(\mathbf{x}) = \underset{j}{\operatorname{argmax}}\, P(\Omega_j | \mathbf{x}),$$

and, using Bayes rule,

$$j^* = \underset{j}{\operatorname{argmax}}\, P(\mathbf{x}|\Omega_j) P(\Omega_j) \tag{3}$$

where $P(f, \Omega_j)$ are the Likelihood Functions (LFs) and $P(\Omega_j)$ are the prior probabilities of the classes. In the rest of the paper we will assume that the prior $P(\Omega_j)$ is the same for all object classes; thus the Bayes classifier (3) simplifies to

$$j^* = \underset{j}{\operatorname{argmax}}\, P(\mathbf{x}|\Omega_j). \tag{4}$$

Many probabilistic appearance-based methods do not model the pdf on raw pixel data, but on features extracted from the original views. The extension of equation (4) to this case is straightforward: consider a set of features $\{h_1^j, h_2^j, ..., h_{n_j}^j\}$, j = 1,...,k, where each feature vector $h_{n_j}^j$ is computed from the image $x_{n_j}^j, h_{n_j}^j = T(x_{n_j}^j)$ $h_{n_j}^j \in G \equiv \Re^m$. The Bayes classifier (4) will be in this case

$$j^* = \underset{j}{\operatorname{argmax}}\, P(\mathbf{h}|\Omega_j) \tag{5}$$

Probabilistic methods for appearance-based visual object recognition have the advantage of being theoretically optimal from the point of view of classification. A major drawback in these approaches is that the functional form of the probability distribution of an object class Ω_j is not known a priori. Assumptions have to be made regarding to the parametric form of the probability distribution, and parameters have to be learned in order to tailor the chosen parametric form to the pattern class represented by the data d_j . Thus, the performance will depend on the goodness of the assumption for the parametric form, and on whether the data set d_j is a sufficient statistic for the pattern class Ω_j and thus, permits us to estimate properly the distribution's parameters.

5 Spin Glass-Markov Random Fields

A possible strategy for modeling the parametric form of the probability function is to use Gibbs distributions within a Markov Random Field framework. MRF provides a probabilistic foundation for modeling spatial interactions on lattice systems or, more generally, on interacting features. It considers each element of the random vector h as the result of a labeling of all the sites representing h, with respect to a given label set. The MRF joint probability distribution is given by

$$P(\mathbf{h}) = \tfrac{1}{Z} \exp(-E(\mathbf{h})), \quad Z = \sum_{\{\mathbf{h}\}} \exp(-E(\mathbf{h})). \tag{6}$$

The normalizing constant Z is called the partition function, and $E(h)$ is the *energy function* $P(\mathbf{h})$ measures the probability of the occurrence of a particular configurations h; the more probable configurations are those with lower energies. Thus, using MRF modeling, eq (4) will become

$$j^* = \underset{j}{\operatorname{argmax}} \, P(\mathbf{h}|\Omega_j) = \underset{j}{\operatorname{argmin}} \, E(\mathbf{h}|\Omega_j) \tag{7}$$

The rest of this Section will review SG-MRFs (Section 4.1) and how they can be derived from results of statistical physics of disordered systems (Section 4.2).

5.1 Spin Glass-Markov Random Fields: Model Definition

Spin Glass-Markov Random Fields (SG-MRFs) [4] are a new class of MRFs which connect SG-like energy functions (mainly the Hopfield one [1]) with Gibbs distributions via a non linear kernel mapping. The resulting model overcomes many difficulties related to the design of fully connected MRFs, and enables us to use the power of kernels in a probabilistic framework. Consider k object classes Ω_1, Ω_2, ..., Ω_k, and for each object a set of n_j data samples, $d_j = \left\{ \mathbf{x}_1^j, \mathbf{x}_2^j, ..., \mathbf{x}_{n_j}^j \right\}$; $j = 1; \dots k.$ We will suppose to extract, from each data sample d_j a set of features $\left\{ \mathbf{h}_1^j, \mathbf{h}_2^j, ..., \mathbf{h}_{n_j}^j \right\}$. For instance, $\mathbf{h}_{n_j}^j$ can be a color histogram computed from $\mathbf{x}_{n_j}^j$. The SG-MRF probability distribution is given by

$$P_{ZSG-MRF}(\mathbf{x}|\Omega_j) = \tfrac{1}{Z} \exp\!\left[-E_{SG-MRF}(\mathbf{x}|\Omega_j) \right], \tag{8}$$

$$Z = \sum_{\{\mathbf{x}\}} \exp\!\left[-E_{SG-MRF}(\mathbf{x}|\Omega_j) \right],$$

with

$$E_{SG-MRF} = -\sum_{\mu=1}^{p_j} \left[K\!\left(\mathbf{x}, \tilde{\mathbf{x}}^\mu\right) \right]^2, \tag{9}$$

where the function $K\left(h, \tilde{h}^{(\mu_j)}\right)$ is a Generalized Gaussian kernel [14]:

$$K(x,y) = \exp\left\{-\rho\, d_{a,b}(x,y)\right\}, \qquad d_{a,b}(x,y) = \sum\left|x_i^a - y_i^a\right|^b \qquad (10)$$

$\left\{\tilde{h}^{(\mu_j)}\right\}_{\mu=1}^{p_j}$, $j \in [1,\kappa]$ are a set of vectors selected (according to a chosen ansatz, [4]) from the training data that we call *prototypes*. The number of prototypes per class must be finite, and they must satisfy the condition:

$$K\left(\tilde{h}^{(i)}, \tilde{h}^{(l)}\right) = 0, \qquad (11)$$

for all $i, l = 1,\dots p_j$, $i \neq l$ and $j = 0,\dots k$. Note that SG-MRFs are defined on features rather than on raw pixels data. The sites are fully connected, which ends in learning the neighborhood system from the training data instead of choosing it heuristically. As we model the probability distribution on feature vectors and not on raw pixels, SG-MRF is not a generative model. Another key characteristic of the model is that in SG-MRF the functional form of the energy is given by construction. This is achieved using results for statistical physics of Spin Glasses. The next Section sketches the theoretical derivation of the model. The interested reader will find a more detailed discussion in [4].

5.2 Spin Glass-Markov Random Fields: Model Derivation

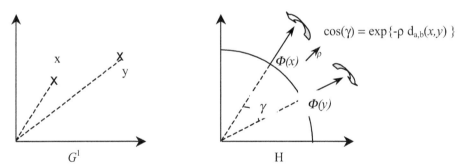

Fig. 2. Gaussian kernels map the data to an infinite dimension hyper-sphere of radius unity. Thus, with a proper choice of ρ, it is possible to orogonalize all the training data in that space

Consider the following energy function:

$$E = -\sum_{(i,j)} J_{ij}\, s_i\, s_j \qquad i,j = 1,2,\dots,N, \qquad (12)$$

where the s_i are random variables taking values in $\{\pm 1\}$, $s = (s_1, \dots, s_N)$ is a configuration and $\mathbf{J} = [J_{ij}]$; $(i; j) = 1, \dots, N$ is the connection matrix, $J_{ij} \in \{\pm 1\}$. Equation (12) is the most general Spin Glass (SG) energy function [1, 9]; the study of the properties of this energy for different Js has been a lively area of research in the statistical physics community for the last 25 years.

An important branch in the research area of statistical physics of SG is represented by the application of this knowledge for modeling brain functions. The simplest and most famous SG model of an associative memory was proposed by Hopfield; it assumes J_{ij} to be given by

$$J_{ij} = \frac{1}{N} \sum_{\mu=1}^{p} \xi_i^{(\mu)} \xi_j^{(\mu)}, \tag{13}$$

where the p sets of $\left\{\xi^{(\mu)}\right\}_{\mu=1}^{p}$ are given configurations of the system (that we call *prototypes*) having the following properties: (a) $\xi^{(\mu)} \perp \xi^{(\nu)}$, $\forall \mu \neq \nu$; (b) $p = \alpha N$, $\alpha \leq 0.14$, $N \to \infty$. Under these assumptions it has been proved that the $\left\{\xi^{(\mu)}\right\}_{\mu=1\_}^{p} = 1$ are the absolute minima of E [1]; for $\alpha > 0.14$ the system loses its storage capability [1]. These results can be extended from the discrete to the continuous case (i.e. s $\in$ [1, +1]^N , see [5]); note that this extension is crucial in the construction of the SG-MRF model.

It is interesting to note that the energy (12), with the prescription (13), can be written as:

$$E = -\frac{1}{N} \sum_{i,j} \sum_{\mu} \xi_i^{(\mu)} \xi_j^{(\mu)} s_i s_j = \frac{1}{N} \sum_{\mu} \left(\xi^{(\mu)} \cdot \mathbf{s}\right)^2 \tag{14}$$

Equation (14) depends on the data through scalar products, thus it can be *kernelized*, as to say it can be written as

$$E_{KAM} = \frac{1}{N} \sum_{\mu} \left(K\left(\xi^{(\mu)} \cdot \mathbf{s}\right)\right)^2. \tag{15}$$

The idea to substitute a kernel function, representing the scalar product in a higher dimensional space, in algorithms depending on just the scalar products between data is the so called *kernel trick* [18], which was first used for Support Vector Machines (SVM); in the last few years theoretical and experimental results have increased the interest within the machine learning and computer vision community regarding the use of kernel functions in methods for classification, regression, clustering, density estimation and so on. We call the energy given by equation (15) Kernel Associative Memory (KAM). KAM energies are of interest in two different research fields: in the formulation given by equation (15) it is a non linear and higher order generalization of the Hopfield energy function. The other research field is computer vision, on which we concentrate the attention here. Indeed, we can look at equation (15) as follows:

$$E = \frac{1}{N} \sum_{\mu} \left(\xi^{(\mu)} \cdot \mathbf{s}\right)^2 = -\frac{1}{N} \sum_{\mu} \left[\Phi\left(\mathbf{h}^{\mu}\right) \cdot \Phi(\mathbf{h})\right]^2 = \frac{1}{N} \sum_{\mu} \left[K\left(\mathbf{h}^{\mu}, \mathbf{h}\right)\right]^2 \tag{16}$$

provided that Φ is a mapping such that (see Figure 1):

$$\Phi : G \equiv \Re \to \infty \, H \equiv [1; +1]^N ; N \to \infty,$$

that in terms of kernel means

$$K(\mathbf{h}, \mathbf{h}) = 1; \ \forall \ \mathbf{h} \in \Re^m; \ dim(H) = N, \ N \rightarrow \infty \qquad (17)$$

If we can find such a kernel, then we can use the KAM energy, with all its properties, for MRF modeling. As the energy is fully connected and the minima of the energy are built by construction, the usage of this energy overcomes all the modeling problems relative to irregular sites for MRF [4]. Conditions (17) are satisfied by generalized Gaussian kernels (10). Regarding the choice of prototypes, given a set of n_k training examples $\{x_1^k, x_2^k, ..., x_{n_k}^k\}$ relative to class Ω_k, the condition to be satisfied by the prototypes is $\xi^{(\mu)} \perp \xi^{(\mu)}$, $\forall \ (\mu \neq \nu)$; in the mapped space H , that becomes $\Phi(h^{(\mu)}) \perp \Phi(h^{(\nu)}) \forall (\mu \neq \nu)$ in the data space G. The measure of the orthogonality of the mapped patterns is the kernel function (10) that, due to the particular properties of Gaussian Kernels, has the effect of orthogonalise the patterns in the space H (see Figure 2). Thus, the orthogonality condition is satisfied by default: if we do not want to introduce further criteria for the choice of prototypes, the natural conclusion is to take all the training samples as prototypes. This approximation is called the naive ansatz.

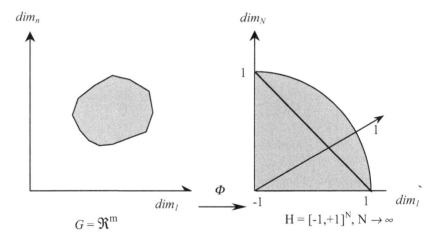

Fig. 3. The kernel trick maps the data from a lower dimension space $G \equiv \Re^m$ to a higher dimension space $H \equiv [-1; +1]^N$; $N \rightarrow \infty$. This permits to use the H-L energy in a MRF framework.

6 Experimental Results

We tested the performance of SG-MRFs for microcalcifications detection on a database of 81 images produced by the "Centro per la Cura e la prevenzione dei Tumori" of the University of Rome "La Sapienza"; each image was digitized from film using a CCD camera operating at a spatial resolution of 604×575 pixels for image; the pixel rate was of 11; 5 MHz, and the pixel size of $10 \mu m \times 15 \ \mu m$. From the 81 images, 152 Region of Interest (ROI) were selected by expert radiologists, each of 128 × 128 pixels. Among the selected 152 ROIs, 112 were positive and 40 were negative; four different ROIs are shown in Figure 1. We used as training set 59 images representing positive ROIs, and 33 images representing negative ROIs. The rest of the database was used as a test set. In a preprocessing step, each extracted ROI was stretched to the normalized gray-level range of 0-255 [6]. Features were extracted using a Multidimensional receptive Field Histogram (MFH) representation [13] 1 , that has been already used successfully combined with SG-MRF [4]. We used 2D MFH, with filters given by Gaussian derivatives along x and y directions as described in Section 2 and with σ = 1.0; resolution for histogram axis of 16 bins. For the classification step, we used SG-MRF in the MAP-MRF framework described in Section 3. For the choice of prototypes, we made a naive ansatz [4], which means that all training views are taken as prototypes, and the ρ in the Gaussian kernel is learned so to satisfy condition (11). The performance of SG-MRF was compared with a Nearest Neighbor Classifier (NNC) and an ANN. More precisely, we used a three-layer perceptron, with backpropagation learning algorithm. the textural features extracted by means of MFH histograms are used as the input signals of the input layer. there is a single output node for classification into positive or negative ROI. The performance of SG-MRF was evaluated as the kernel parameters a; b varied. The performance of the ANN was evaluated as the number of neurons in the hidden layer varied. NNC SG-MRF ANN

Table 1. Classification results for NNC, ANN and SG-MRF. S1 represents the number of neurons in the hidden layer for ANN.

NNC	SG-MRF				ANN			
	a = 1, b = 1.5	88.33	a = 0.5, b = 1.5	93.33	S_1=1	83.33	S_1=4	83.33
88.33	a = 1, b = 1	90.00	a = 0.5, b = 1	93.33	S_1=2	83.33	S_1=5	83.33

Classification results are reported in Table 1. The best recognition rate, corresponding to 93.33%, was obtained using SG-MRF. This result is obtained with more than one combination of kernel parameters (see Table 1). NNC gives a best performance of 88.33%, corresponding to a +5% less with respect to the recognition rate obtained using SG-MRF. ANN gives a best performance of 85.00%, corresponding to the worst recognition rate obtained on this database. It corresponds to a 3.33% loss with respect to the recognition rate obtained using NNC, and to an impressive 8.33% loss with respect to the recognition rate obtained using SG-MRF. 1 We gratefully thank B. Schiele who allowed us to use his software for the computation of MFH. These results show the effectiveness of SG-MRF for microcalcification detection. At the same time, they show that, in the building of algorithms for computer-assisted diagnosis, ANN cannot be considered a priori the optimal choice for the classification step. To the best of our knowledge, these are the first experiments that reports of a comparative study on microcalcification detection with respect to the kind of classifier employed.

7 Summary

In this paper we presented a new probabilistic approach for microcalcification detection. It applies a new kernel method, Spin Glass-Markov Random Fields, that already proved to be very effective for many visual applications such as object recognition and scene classification [4]. The method is benchmarked with a NNC and an ANN on the same feature representation, obtaining respectively an impressive +5% and +8.33% recognition rate. This experimental result shows the effectiveness of the proposed approach. This work can be extended in many ways. First, the performance of SG-MRF can be improved choosing a different set of kernel parameters, and a different representation. Second, we plan to benchmark this approach with other classifiers such as support vector machines. Finally, we intend to compare the performance of SG-MRF and the aforementioned classifiers using different set of features. Future work will concentrate in these directions.

Acknowledgments We would like to thank Prof. V. Virno and the staff of the Radiology department of the "Centro per la cura e la Prevenzione dei Tumori" of the University of Rome "La Sapienza". B. C. has been supported by the Foundation BLANCEFLOR Boncompagni-Ludovisi.

References

1. D. J. Amit, "Modeling Brain Function", Cambridge University Press, 1989.
2. C. M. Bishop, Neural Networks for Pattern Recognition, Claredon Press - Oxford, 1995.
3. B. Caputo, G. E. Gigante, "Digital Mammography: a Weak Continuity Texture Representation for Detection of Microcalcifications", Proc. of SPIE Medical Imaging 2001, February 17-22, VOL 4322, PP1705-1716, San Diego, (CA), USA, 2001.
4. B. Caputo, H. Niemann, "From Markov Random Fields to Associative Memories and Back: Spin Glass Markov Random Fields", SCTV2001.
5. J. J. Hopfield, "Neurons with graded response have collective computational properties like those of two-state neurons", Proc. Natl. Acad. Sci. USA, Vol. 81, pp 30883092, 1984.
6. A. K. Jain, "Fundamental of digital image processing", Prentice Hall, Englewood Cliffs, 1989.
7. M. Lanyi, "Diagnosis and Differential Diagnosis of Breast Calcifications", New York: Springer-Verlag, 1986.
8. R. P. Lippmann, "An introduction to computing with neural nets", IEEE ASSP Magazine, pp. 4-22, April 1987.
9. M. Mezard, G. Parisi, M. Virasoro, "Spin Glass Theory and Beyond", World Scientific, Singapore, 1987.
10. S. Morio and S. Kawahara et al., "Expert system for early detection of cancer of the breast", Comp. Biol. Med., vol. 19, no. 5, pp. 295-305, 1989.
11. Nishikawa RM, Wolverton DE, Schmidt RA, Papaioannou J, "Radiologists' ability to discriminate computer-detected true and false positives, from an automated scheme for the detection of clustered microcalcifications on digital mammograms", Proc SPIE 3036: 198-204, 1997.
12. D. E. Rumelhart and C.R. Rosemberg, Parallel Distributed Processing, the MIT Press, Cambridge MA, 1986.

13. B. Schiele, J. L. Crowley, "Recognition without correspondence using multidimensional receptive field histograms",IJCV, 36 (1), pp. 31- 52, 2000.
14. B. Schölkopf, A. J. Smola, Learning with kernels, 2001, the MIT Press.
15. L.Shen, R. M. Rangayyan and J. E. L. Desautels, "Application of shape analysis to mammographic calcifications", IEEE Trans. Med Imag., vol. 13, no. 2, pp. 263-274, 1994.
16. E. A. Sickles and D. B. Kopans, "Mammographic screening for women aged 40 to 49 years: the primary practitioner's dilemma", Anna. Intern. Med., vol. 122, no. 7, pp. 534-538, 1995.
17. M. Swain, D. Ballard, "color Indexing", IJCV, 7, pp 11-32, 1991.
18. V. Vapnik, Statistical learning theory, J. Wiley, New York, 1998.
19. Zhang W, Doi K, Giger ML, Nishikawa RM, Schmidt RA, "An improved shift - invariant artificial neural network for computerized detection of clustered microcalcifications in digital mammograms". Med Phys, 23: 595-601, 1996.

The Use of Classification Trees for Analysis of Kidney Images in Computer Assisted Microscopy

Elzbieta Kaczmarek, Edyta Nieruchalska, Michal Michalak, Aldona Wozniak, and Wieslawa Salwa-Zurawska

Lab. of Morphometry and Medical Image Processing,
Chair and Department of Pathomorphology, Karol Marcinkowski University of Medical Sciences, 60-355 Poznan, Przybyszewskiego 49

Abstract. The aim of this paper is to present an application of classification trees for quantitative analysis of kidney specimens in light and electron microscopy. Minimal change disease (MCD) cases, focal segmental glomerulosclerosis (FSGS) cases, and mesangial glomerulonephritis cases suspected of being progressive into MCD or FSGS were analysed in our study. At first, fuzzy logic was applied for processing and segmentation of structures in colour and grey scale images. Glomerular profiles, interstitial fibrosis and normal part of interstitium were segmented from colour light micrographs and then their area was estimated. The volume of glomerular mesangium, matrix and cell components were assessed in electron micrographs. These measurements were selected as predictor variables for classification trees. Results of classification presented in this paper indicated that the medical diagnosis of certain glomerulopathies should be performed in light and electron microscopy. The ratio of matrix volume to the whole mesangium determined in electron microscopy and the mean glomerular area estimated in light microscopy are the most important features for diagnosis of suspected cases as MCD or early phase of FSGS cases.

1   Introduction

Morphological changes of renal glomeruli and/or interstitial fibrosis appear in process of several kidney diseases. In normal cases, light microscopy (LM) images of kidney show networks of thin blue fibres spanning in red interstitium and around renal glomeruli. In process of formation of interstitial fibrosis, blue area expands and the area of renal glomeruli cross sections often changes [3]. Light microscopy of first biopsy specimen frequently does not reveal the increase of matrix inside renal glomeruli, although is generally detected in electron microscopy (EM). Therefore, cases diagnosed as minimal change disease (MCD), focal segmental glomerulosclerosis (FSGS), mesangial glomerulonephritis suspected of being progressing into FSGS and MCD cases suspected of being progressing into mesangial glomerulonephritis ('suspected cases') were analysed in our study. To support medical decision, all cases were investigated in light and electron microscopy. After image processing, renal glomeruli and interstitial fibrosis were segmented and quantified in LM images while matrix, mesangium and cellular components were segmented and quantified in EM images.

A. Colosimo et al. (Eds.): ISMDA 2002, LNCS 2526, pp. 32–41, 2002.

The aim of this paper is to present an application of classification trees for medical diagnosis of certain kidney diseases on the basis of selected morphometric parameters determined in computer assisted microscopy.

2   Image Acquisition

Kidney biopsies of 47 children were subjects of quantitative light microscopy studies. Kidney images were registered with a computer-assisted light microscope. Each colour image of 760x570 pixels (24 bits per pixel) was recorded and stored by using image analysis system MicroImage v.4.0 (Olympus).

Electron micrographs (1280x1024 pixels, 12 bits) were taken for quantitative image analysis in 256 grey scale tones. Usually 10-20 colour light micrographs and 10 electron micrographs showing the most severe changes of the mesangial area were acquired per each case.

3   Image Analysis

Colour images of interstitium were first smoothed by using the averaging approach within a 3x3 sample matrix of pixels to remove noisy pixels. Interstitial fibrosis (blue tones) was defined in three intervals of RGB coordinates: R=(45; 75), G=(105; 155) and B=(140; 180). The remaining colours represented the normal part of interstitium (red tones). Then, colour contrast between two pixels was defined as the squared value of the Euclidean distance between the colour vectors $v_i=(R_i, G_i, B_i)$ and $v_j=(R_j, G_j, B_j)$. The contrast between the two colour vectors: $v_{light\_blue}=(45, 105, 140)$ and $v_{dark\_blue}=(75, 155, 180)$ was the threshold for blue tones.

Colour contrast between a pixel and the average colour of its eight neighbours was then calculated and compared with the threshold for blue tones. If the contrast at one direction exceeded the threshold value then the pixel colour was decided to belong to red tones else to blue tones. Thus, edges between red normal interstitium and blue interstitial fibrosis were detected [3].

A light microscopy image of kidney specimen (Fig. 1 a) shows the interstitial fibrosis (in blue colours) and the result of its segmentation (Fig. 1d). To get the final result, two classes of blue tones (light and dark) representing the fibrosis (Fig. 2) were segmented and combined by the union ("OR") operation (Fig. 1d).

Electron micrographs (grey scale images) were processed by a mean filter to reduce the noise (in case of need). Moreover, brightness normalisation was performed on the basis of histogram extremes of an image that was chosen as a reference image. Thus, all processed electron micrographs were converted into images of comparable brightness and contrast levels.

To segment mesangium, mesangial matrix and cell components from EM images, the intervals of grey levels representing these structures were defined [4].

The analysed structures, i.e. matrix, mesangium and cell components, were segmented by using fuzzy logic algorithms [4] for the following classes of pixels:

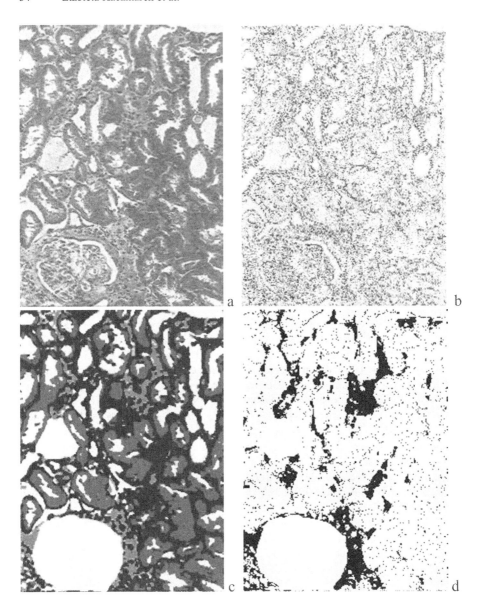

Fig. 1. A llight microscopy image of kidney specimen with three renal glomeruli (a), the effect of image smoothing (b), the result of thresholding of smoothed image with removed profiles of renal glomeruli (c), and the segmented interstitial fibrosis (d).

'background' – intervals of grey levels corresponding with the general scene against which the analysed structures were viewed,

'interior' - intervals of grey levels as inside the extracted structures,

'outer neighbourhood' - intervals of grey levels as in the nearest neighbourhood surrounding the extracted structures.

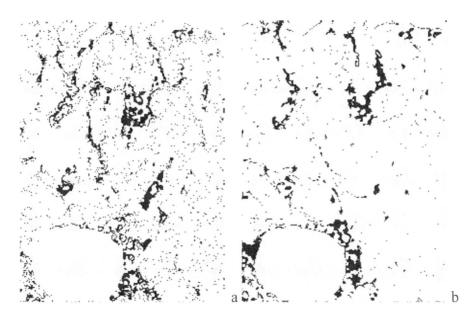

Fig. 2. Segmentation of interstitial fibrosis: dark blue area (a) segmented from the thresholded image (Fig. 1c) and light blue area (b) segmented from the same image. The result of OR operator for images (a) and (b) is shown in Fig. 1d.

Then, IF-THEN fuzzy rules were defined. For instance:
    IF pixel x_i belongs to *'background'* AND pixel x_j belongs
        to *'outer neighbourhood'*   THEN   set colour of the pixel x_j as *'black'*;
    IF x_i belongs to *'outer neighbourhood'* AND pixel x_j belongs to *'interior'*
        THEN   set colour of the pixel x_i as *'white'*.

All cases analysed in this study were first evaluated by a pathologist and diagnosed as MCD cases (16 patients) and FSGS cases (11 patients). Mesangial glomerulonephritis cases suspected of being progressing into FSGS and MCD cases suspected of being progressing into mesangial glomerulonephritis were assigned to the same group named „suspected cases" (20 patients).

Each case was quantitatively assessed in 15-20 light microscopy images and 5 electron microscopy images selected by pathologists. In each LM image, the area of interstitial fibrosis and the remaining area of the image were measured. The degree of fibrosis was assessed as the ratio of the total area of interstitial fibrosis determined in all images of the same case to the total remaining area of the same images with previously removed glomerular profiles [3]. Then, the mean glomerular area per case was computed. For the same case (patient), the total area of matrix (Mat), the total area of mesangium (Mes) and the total area of cellular components (Cell) were determined in electron micrographs. Then, the ratios Mat/Mes and Mat/Cell were calculated [8], [9].

4   Application of Classification Trees

4.1 Computational Methods

In this paper, binary classification trees were determined based on univariate splits for predictor variables. The split selection method was the C&RT-style exhaustive search. With the C&RT-style exhaustive search method all possible splits for each predictor variable at each node were examined to find the split producing the largest improvement in goodness of fit. Goodness of fit was used as criterion for selecting the best split from the set of possible candidate splits.

The improvement in goodness of fit can be determined by the Gini measure of node impurity, the chi-square measure or G-square measure.

The Gini measure is computed as the sum of products of all pairs of class proportions for classes present at the node. It reaches its maximum value when class sizes at the node are equal while a value of zero when only one class is present at a node (with priors estimated from class sizes and equal misclassification costs).

The chi-square measure was derived from the Chi-square distribution defined by:

$$f(x) = \{1/[2v/2* \Gamma(v/2)]\} * [x(v/2)\text{-}1 * e\text{-}x/2], \qquad n = 1, 2, \dots \text{ and } x > 0 \qquad (11)$$

where v is the degrees of freedom,
            e is the base of the natural logarithm,
            Γ (gamma) is the Gamma function.

The G-square measure was computed as the maximum likelihood Chi-square [1], [6].

For the criterion variable, pruning of the tree can be based on misclassification errors. We can specify the maximum number of nodes for the tree or the minimum group size per node. In this paper, we decided to specify the minimum group size. For validating the best decision tree, we used V-fold cross validation.

4.2 Application

In our study, the binary classification trees were determined to predict membership of cases in the classes of a categorical dependent variable DIAGNOSIS (MCD, FSGS and 'SUSPECTED' cases) from their measurements on the predictor variables (mean glomerular area, degree of interstitial fibrosis, Mat/Mes, Mat/Cell) converted into ordinal scales of ranks. The split selection method was the C&RT-style exhaustive search assuming that the smallest group size was 5. The improvement in goodness of fit was determined by the Gini measure, chi-square and G-square measures and then compared. For the test sample cross-validation, the classification tree was computed from the learning sample, and its predictive accuracy was tested by applying it to predict class membership in the test sample. If the costs for the test sample exceeded the costs for the learning sample, this indicated poor cross-validation and that a different sized tree might cross-validate better.

5   Results

The C&RT method for mean glomerular area, degree of interstitial fibrosis, Mat/Mes, Mat/Cell as predictors correctly classified 41 of the 47 cases (87.2 %).

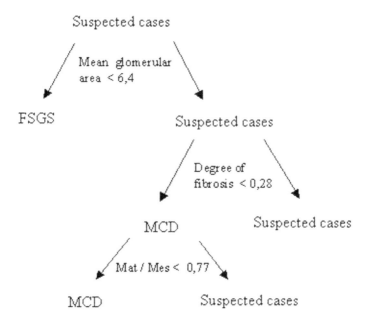

Fig. 3. Classification tree for mean glomerular area, degree of interstitial fibrosis, and ratios Mat/Mes, Mat/Cell as predictors.

The results of classification obtained with Gini, chi-square and G-square measures were the same. The classification tree (Fig. 3) assigned suspected cases into FSGS group if mean glomerular area was lower than 6,4 micron^2. 'Suspected' cases with larger glomeruli were assigned to MCD group if the degree of fibrosis was lower than 0,28 and Mat/Mes < 0,77 otherwise the cases belonged to the 'suspected' group of mesangial glomerulonephritis cases (GnMES) cases.

The cross validation cost calculated for the classification tree computed from the learning sample exceeded the cost for the test sample for each used measure of goodness of fit (Table 1).

Table 1. Cross-validation costs for the classification trees

Goodness of fit	Cross-validation for the tree	Cross-validation for the test sample
Gini measure	0,43	0,36
Chi-square measure	0,27	0,09
G-square measure	0,19	0,09

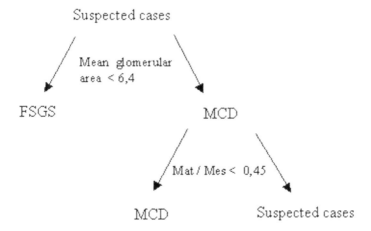

Fig. 4. Classification tree for mean glomerular area and ratios Mat/Mes, Mat/Cell as predictors.

Predictor variable importance rankings for dependent variable DIAGNOSIS showed rather high importance of all variables. However, the ratio Mat/Mes showed the highest rank 100 while the degree of fibrosis had the lowest rank 81% (Fig. 5).

Since the degree of fibrosis showed the lowest rank of importance, we performed another classification based on predictors describing only renal glomeruli, i.e. mean glomerular area, Mat/Mes, Mat/Cell and the same dependent variable DIAGNOSIS. The classification tree (Fig. 4) assigned suspected cases into FSGS group if mean glomerular area was lower than 6,4 micron^2. 'Suspected' cases with larger glomeruli were assigned to MCD group if Mat/Mes<0,45 otherwise the cases belonged to the 'suspected' group of mesangial glomerulonephritis (GnMES) cases. Only one case was misclassified.

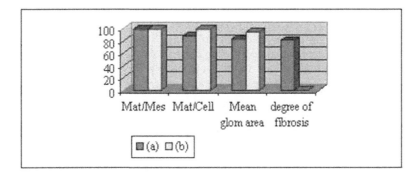

Fig. 5. The importance ranks of degree of fibrosis and glomerular features as predictors (a), and exclusively glomerular features as predictors (b).

Table 2. Morphometric features of the analysed cases

Group	Feature	Mean	S. D.	Min	Max
MCD	Mat/Cell	1,01	1,17	0,24	4,44
	Mat/Mes	0,41	0,18	0,20	0,82
	Mean glom. area	13,81	4,84	6,05	21,87
	degree of fibrosis	0,22	0,07	0,12	0,37
FSGS	Mat/Cell	1,32	0,36	1,07	1,94
	Mat/Mes	0,56	0,06	0,52	0,66
	Mean glom. area	14,24	8,10	7,29	29,09
	degree of fibrosis	0,43	0,16	0,23	0,76
'suspected' cases	Mat/Cell	1,73	1,03	1,01	5,00
	Mat/Mes	0,61	0,09	0,50	0,83
	Mean glom. area	25,22	10,36	12,07	50,48
	degree of fibrosis	0,36	0,12	0,14	0,68

The cross validation cost computed from the learning sample was 0,238 and exceeded the cost for the test sample 0,045. Predictor variable importance rankings for the variable DIAGNOSIS showed the highest importance of electron micrographs' features of renal glomeruli (Mat/Mes and Mat/Cell). However, the importance rank of the mean glomerular area evaluated in LM images was also very high (Fig. 5). The summary statistics of morphometric features of studied groups is shown in Table 2.

6 Discussion

Feature extraction and classification are the crucial steps in pattern recognition [5], [7]. The classification procedure can be simplified as a transformation of quantitative input data to qualitative output information. The statistical methods and neural networks can use the same features. However neural networks require large data sets for the appropriate results of classification. Neural networks may be characterised by their learning process. Supervised learning algorithms require the exemplary data set to be classified before the training task [5]. Our data set is not large enough for this purpose.

In clustering, the existence of predefined patterns is not assumed, the number of clusters or the class membership can be unknown. The task of clustering process is to group the features to clusters in which the similarity of patterns is stronger than between the clusters. The area fractions in evaluated images (degree of fibrosis, Mat/Mes, Mat/Cell) and the mean glomerular area, which might be related with the progress of the studied diseases, were extracted and analysed in our study. Thus, values of the measurement scales of the features were quite various and caused unsatisfactory results of clustering for a variety of distance functions (one large cluster of cases and some one-element clusters or a number of small size clusters).

Therefore, we decided to convert the original measurement scales of data into ordinal scales of ranks and use classification trees. Without using any prior knowledge of the values for the predictor variables, that a case will fall into one of the classes, we estimated prior probabilities that the likelihood that a case or object will fall into one of the classes is proportional to the dependent variable class sizes.

For classification problems, various measures can be chosen to modify the algorithm and to evaluate the quality of the final classification tree by specifying prior classification probabilities and misclassification costs. However, the Gini measure was the measure of goodness of fit preferred by the developers of C&RT method [2].

At present, we are not able to state that the more accurate classification is desired for some classes than others. Therefore, it is difficult to specify misclassification costs which can be used to weight the analysis more heavily toward some classes than for others. This is why we assume equal costs of misclassifying objects in an observed class as belonging to another class. Thus, in our study, each off-diagonal element of the predicted class (row) x observed class (column) of misclassification costs matrix is set equal to 1.0 .

The results obtained with classification trees based on three measures of goodness of fit were rather consistent with a preliminary qualitative classification made by pathologists.

Our earlier results based on electron microscopy studies of glomerulopathies indicated that the ratios Mat/Mes and Mat/Cell were linearly correlated in children with MCD, FSGS and GnMes [8], [9]. Moreover, Mat/Mes<0.5 and Mat/Cell<1.0 for MCD cases while for FSGS cases Mat/Mes>0.5 and Mat/Cell>1.0 [8], [9]. The mentioned results are consistent with the results presented in this paper.

In contrast to our earlier studies, classification trees allowed us to support medical decision based on multivariate analysis of features segmented from both light and electron micrographs. Feature importance ranking and classification tree plot indicate that the degree of fibrosis is not necessarily related with morphological changes of renal glomeruli observed in light and electron microscopy.

References

1. Bain, L. J. and Engelhart, M., Introduction to Probability and Mathematical Statistics. PWS, Kent, MA. (1989).
2. Breiman, L., Friedman, J. H., Olshen, R. A., & Stone, C. J., Classification and regression trees. Monterey, CA, Wadsworth & Brooks/Cole Advanced Books & Software (1984).
3. Kaczmarek E., Wozniak A., Salwa-Zurawska W., Fuzzy Sets Applied to Image Processing and Quantification of Interstitial Fibrosis and Glomerular Size in Computer Assisted Microscopy. In: Medical Data Analysis, J. Crespo, V. Maojo, F. Martin (Eds.), LNCS 2199, Springer Verlag 2001, 120-125.
4. Kaczmarek E: Fuzzy logic for image processing and analysis of renal glomeruli observed in light, confocal and electron microscopes. In: Image Processing III. Mathematical Methods, Algorithms and Applications. J.M. Blackledge & M.J. Turnes (Eds.). Horwood Publishing Series: Mathematics and Applications, Chichester 2001, 102-112.
5. Leondes C.T. (Ed.), Image Processing and Pattern Recognition. Academic Press, London, New York (1998).
6. Neter, J., Wasserman, W., & Kutner, M. H., Applied linear regression models (2nd ed.). Homewood, IL: Irwin. (1989).
7. Russ J.C., Computer Assisted Microscopy. The Measurement and Analysis of Images. Plenum, New York, third edition (1992).

8. Wozniak A., Salwa-Zurawska W., Kaczmarek E., Bortkiewicz E., Gladysz J., Maciejewski J., The Application of Electron Microscopy Morphometry as Helpful Method in the Diagnosis of Focal Segmental Glomerulosclerosis (FSGS) Early Phase I. Morphometric Electron Microscopic Studies of Renal Glomeruli in Cases of Focal Segmental Glomerulosclerosis (FSGS), Minimal Change Disease (MCD) and Mesagioproloferative Glomerulonephritis (GNMES) in Children. Pol. J. Pathol. 2001, Vol. 52 (1-2): 27-36.

9. Wozniak A., Bortkiewicz E., Salwa-Zurawska W., Kaczmarek E., Maciejewski J., The Application of Electron Microscopy Morphometry as Helpful Method in the Diagnosis of Focal Segmental Glomerulosclerosis (FSGS) Early Phase. II. Clinical Usefulness of Electron Microscopic Morphometric Studies in Cases of Focal Segmental Glomerulosclerosis (FSGS), Minimal Change Disease (MCD) and Mesagioproloferative Glomerulonephritis (GNMES) with Suspicion of Progression into Focal Segmental Glomerulosclerosis (FSGS). Pol. J. Pathol. 2001, Vol. 52 (1-2): 37-46.

A Neuro-fuzzy Based Alarm System for Septic Shock Patients with a Comparison to Medical Scores

Jürgen Paetz[1,2] and Björn Arlt[1,2]

[1] J.W. Goethe-Universität Frankfurt am Main,
Fachbereich Biologie und Informatik,
Institut für Informatik, AG Adaptive Systemarchitektur
Robert-Mayer-Straße 11-15, D-60054 Frankfurt am Main, Germany
[2] Klinikum der J.W. Goethe-Universität,
Klinik für Allgemein- und Gefäßchirurgie
Theodor-Stern-Kai 7, D-60590 Frankfurt am Main, Germany
{paetz,arlt}@cs.uni-frankfurt.de
http://www.medan.de

Abstract During the last years we collected data of abdominal *septic shock* patients from clinics all over Germany. The mortality of septic shock is about 50%. Septic shock is related to immune system reactions and unusual measurements. Septic shock patients are intensely medicated during their stay at the intensive care unit. To help physicians recognizing the critical states of their patients as early as possible, we built a *rule based alarm system* based on a neuro-fuzzy inference machine. Analysing the patient data in a time window, we show the time dependency of the classification results. We give detailed classification results and explanation by rules. The results are compared to results obtained by using the most common *scores* in intensive care medicine. We discuss the advantages of the paradigms "neural networks" and "scores", and we answer the important question: Is a neural network more performant than scores for abdominal septic shock patient data?

1   Introduction

Septic shock is of prime importance in intensive care medicine. Epidemiologic investigations of septic shock patients show the high risk potential and the extensive therapy situation in intensive care units (ICU) [1]. Variables are often investigated as isolated variables, not as a multidimensional whole, e.g. a recent study inspects the role of thrombocytes [2].

Our approach to reduce mortality of septic shock patients is the automated, intelligent retrospective search of information in documented patient records. We analysed the data of 138 patients by using most of the usually documented metric variables (e.g. blood pressure, leukocytes, medicament doses). Data was collected in German hospitals from 1998 to 2001. Up to now we have digitized 138 collected handwritten patient records. 70 of the 138 patients are deceased

A. Colosimo et al. (Eds.): ISMDA 2002, LNCS 2526, pp. 42–52, 2002.

(50.7%). Our analysis of metric data carries on the analyses already done with another data base and other methods, e.g. [3]. The scores that are often used in the ICU are described in Sect. 2. To find interesting rules within the high number of all the rules coming from subsets of all the variables we used a neuro-fuzzy algorithm based on [4,5] which is described in Sect. 3. Subsequently, in Sect. 4 achieved results are presented. We compare the scoring results to the neuro-fuzzy results, and we give some meaningful rule examples. The results culminate in an alarm system whose performance is analysed.

2   Scores in Intensive Care Medicine

How could physicians assess the patient's health status as objectively as possible? An easy practiced method is to model expert opinions by using a *score*, i.e. a sum of points. This action is not fully objective, but it represents joint expert opinions. By defining a threshold the score can be utilized as a classifier for outcome prediction. We present shortly the most common scores used in intensive care medicine. Classification results of applied scores are given in Sect. 4.4.

a) *SOFA* (Sepsis-Related Organ Failure Assessment) [7]: the SOFA score assesses organ malfunctions by whole-numbered values. The sum of these values for the single organs is called SOFA score.

b) *APACHE II* (Acute Physiological and Chronic Health Evaluation) [8]: APACHE II is a score for outcome prognosis of ICU patients with respect to acute disorders, age and the overall health status (0 to 71 whole-numbered points).

c) *SAPS II* (Simplified Acute Physiology Score) [9]: The SAPS II score is a variable reduced APACHE II score. Only 13 instead of 34 variables are used.

d) *MODS* (Multiple Organ Dysfunction Score) [10]: The MODS score assesses organ states (lungs, liver, kidney, haemogram, heart, neurological system) by whole-numbered points.

In the SOFA and MODS score we do not include the Glasgow Coma Scale (GCS) for assessing the neurological state because of its impreciseness and its high subjectivity.

3   The Neuro-fuzzy System

The supervised neuro-fuzzy algorithm [4] uses the class information of the data within its adaptation process. Here, we use the outcome labels "survived" and "deceased" for the classes. The main advantages of the algorithm are:

- The training uses a simple heuristic geometric adaptation process that softens the combinatorical explosion (exponential growth) during the rule generation process due to multiple dimensions.
- Irrelevant attributes for every rule are detected. This is the case if a part of a rule R has the format "**if** ... **and** var$_j$ **in** $(-\infty, +\infty)$ **and** ... **then** class ...". Then, the value of variable j is not relevant and so the variable could be omitted, leading to a shorter rule R.
- Adaptive learning of the exact shape of the trapezoid membership functions.

Let us describe the ideas of the algorithm. The 2-layer neural network has neurons in the hidden layer with n-dimensional asymmetrical trapezoidal fuzzy activation functions. Every neuron in the first layer belongs to only one class and represents a fuzzy rule. During the learning phase these neurons p are adapted, i.e. the sides of the upper, smaller rectangles (= *core rules*) and the sides of the lower, larger rectangles (= *support rules*) of the trapezoids are adapted to the data. For every new training data point x of class c this happens in four phases, initialized by the first training sample x_1 for which one neuron is committed with infinite side expansions in every dimension for the support rule and no (zero) expansion for the core rule (core rule = x_1):

1. *cover*: if x lies in the region of a support rule of the same class c as x, expand one side of the corresponding core rule to cover x and increment the weight of the neuron,
2. *commit*: if no such support rule covers x, insert a new neuron p at point x of the same class and set its weight to one and its center $z := x$. The expansions of the sides of the support rule – associated with the new neuron – are set to infinite; the expansions of the sides of the core rule – associated with the new neuron – are set to zero,
3. *shrink committed neuron*: for a committed neuron shrink the volume of the support (and the core rectangle if necessary) within one heuristically chosen dimension of the neuron in relation to the neurons belonging to other classes,
4. *shrink conflict neurons*: for all the neurons belonging to another class $\neq c$, heuristically shrink the volume of both rectangles of these neurons within one dimension in relation to x.

A sketch of the standard algorithm [4] is given in Appendix A. For implementation details of our more technical modifications and improvements see [5,6]. Here, we place emphasis on the application to our septic shock patient data.

4   Results

At first we give a short description of the database and the datasets. Then, we present the experimental conditions and the classification results of the neurofuzzy and score classifiers with a discussion. Meaningful rule examples are presented.

4.1   The Datasets

Our database consists of 138 septic shock patients. The metric data that we consider is composed of daily measurements and doses of medicaments. For the experiments that are presented in Fig. 1, we consider different *periods of time*: F3 (first 3 days of ICU stay), S3 (first 3 days after the septic shock occurence), ALL (all days of ICU stay), D6–8 (days 6,7 and 8 counted from the last day, i.e. day 0, of ICU stay), D2–4 (days 2,3 and 4 counted from the last day of ICU stay), L5, L3, L2, L1 (last 5 resp. 3, 2, 1 day(s) of ICU stay). In Figs. 2 and 3 we regard only the period L3, cf. the explanation in Sect. 4.3.

We consider the following datasets in our contribution: frequent16 (the most frequent 16 measured variables), haemogram, heart, lungs, bac (breathing and catecholamines), bpt (systolic and diastolic blood pressure, thrombocytes) and the single variables systolic blood pressure, diastolic blood pressure, thrombocytes, see appendix B for more details.

Here, we will mention only our main preprocessing steps [3]: sampling (mean values of 24h) and missing value removal (missing values are replaced by random values from a normal distribution within the interval of the so called interquartile range, abbr. IQR, with the median as the center).

4.2 Experimental Conditions

All the samples of the datasets are classified by the neuro-fuzzy system. Training was done with 50% of the samples and testing with the remaining 50%. No data from training patients is used for testing (disjunct patient sets). All experiments with one dataset were repeated five times, so that all given results are average values of all experiments. Thus, random results are avoided.

To compare classification performance, we use the area under the ROC curve (AUC). The ROC curve is given by sensitivity values on y-axis and specifity values on x-axis. It is equal to 0.5 if the classifier has no performance (random classification) and equal to 1.0 if the classifier performs without errors. Here, each ROC curve is calculated using 10 different classification thresholds, i.e. sensitivity/specifity settings. The AUC is calculated with the well known trapeze rule for numerical integration.

4.3 Neuro-fuzzy-System Performance

The best outcome predictor would be one that warns the physician at the first day of ICU admission or at the first day of septic shock appearance (that is mostly the second day of the patient's ICU stay). With the dataset "frequent16" we show in Fig. 1 that it is not possible to train an adequate prediction system within such an early time interval (F3 AUC = 0.53, S3 AUC = 0.58). Also it is not reliable to base the system on the samples of *all* days (ALL AUC = 0.67). Unfortunately, within the last two days often less samples are measured by physicians so that the results considering L2 and L1 are not trusting or significant. The best classification results are achieved considering L3 (AUC = 0.92). Thus, in the following we consider only the period L3.

The results achieved with the dataset "frequent16" (period L3) are encouraging, but it is not reliable for physicians to key in 16 variables. The SOFA score is based only on 10 variables. Is it possible to achieve a similar performance using less variables? To answer this question, we tried out different compositions of variables. The results are presented in Fig. 2. We see that single variables have not a sufficient performance. The best performance is achieved by the haemogram (AUC = 0.90) and by "frequent16" (AUC = 0.92). As said before keying in 14 resp. 16 variables in an alarm system is too much. Thus, the system "bpt" (3 variables) with an equal AUC = 0.90 is a good candidate for building an alarm system, but only if it performs not worse than the established scores, cf. the next section.

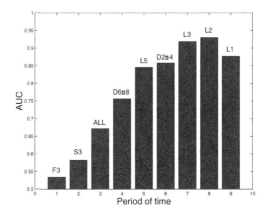

Figure 1. "Frequent16" data: Area under ROC curve (AUC) for different periods of time of the ICU stay.

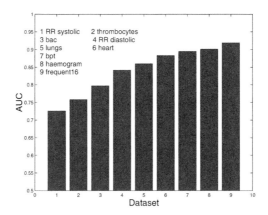

Figure 2. Area under ROC curve (AUC) for different data sets (last three days of ICU stay).

4.4   Score Performance

In Fig. 3 we see that the three scores MODS, SAPS II and APACHE II perform almost equally well (AUC = 0.79 , 0.79 resp. 0.80), considering the time period

L3. We achieve an obvious better classification using the SOFA score (AUC = 0.89). The SOFA score, that is composed of 10 variables, does not perform better than the "bpt" or "frequent16" system. Therefore, it could be replaced in the ICU by using an alarm system whose alarm behaviour is described in Sect. 4.6.

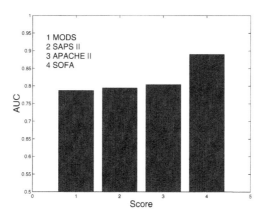

Figure 3. Area under ROC curve (AUC) for the scores MODS, SAPS II, APA-CHE II and SOFA.

One question remains open: Why is the adaptive data driven neural network approach not *much* more performant than a "simple" score? Firstly, only one score – the SOFA score – has a similar performance. Secondly, the SOFA score was evaluated on 1643 patients in the USA (more than 10 times the number of patients that we consider), surely including many expert opinions or even statistical methods. Thirdly, our analyses are retrospective analyses with a lower quality as potential prospective analyses due to missing values.

Without presenting all the details of our analysis, the results of a binary logistic regression, using SPSS 9.0, are very similar to the results achieved by our rule-based system. Thus, binary logistic regression is also not much more performant than the SOFA score on our data.

Finally, the SOFA score is computed somewhat similar to a neural network output: 1 up to 4 points are given individually for every variable state by a nonlinear, discrete step function. Then, these values are added up. In a neural network the activities of the neurons in the first layer are added up in the second layer. Of course, the neural network learns its activities by a data driven training autonomously. This would give better results as a score if and only if the step functions within a score are chosen badly. Thus, it seems that the step functions in the SOFA score are chosen well. If our data would have more complex, nonlinear class borders, a neural network approach would surely give much better results since then one cannot guess correct classification without a machine learning approach, even not by investing a lot of time for trial and error based data analysis. Inventing a score without using a machine learning approach is experience based trial and error data analysis, hoping to obtain good results.

To sum up, we cannot beat sigificantly the SOFA score's performance by our approach (or by binary logistic regression without rule generation), but we are able to reduce the number of variables and give important insight by our rules. We need three variables only for our alarm system instead of ten variables used for calculation of the SOFA score. It seems that the variables in the "bpt" system are the "core" variables whose trends are common to most of the patients. The use of additional variables in the other systems seems to be more influenced by individual patient behaviour with less performant classification results. Besides the "bpt" system, a mixture of variables from different systems as in the "frequent16" system or in the SOFA score give good results.

4.5   Generated Rules

We present the results of our rule generation for the dataset "bpt". On average we generated 7.6 rules for the class "deceased" and 8.2 for the class "survived". To evaluate the performance of the rules we calculated the frequency (percentage of all samples that imply the rule) and the confidence (percentage of samples of the correct class considering all samples that imply the rule) of the rules on the test data. Let us give two important examples of frequent and confident (support) rules:

1) class **survived** with frequency $= 30.5\%$ and confidence $= 98.4\%$ if
systolic blood pressure ≥ 111.8 and
diastolic blood pressure ≥ 41.7 and
thrombocytes in $(264.0,700.0)$

2) class **deceased** with frequency $= 40.5\%$ and confidence $= 91.4\%$ if
systolic blood pressure ≤ 127.5 and
diastolic blood pressure ≤ 62.8 and
thrombocytes ≤ 282.0

These rules show that a lower systolic and diastolic blood pressure and a lower number of thrombocytes indicate very critical diseasedness. Quantified results as the results above may lead to more precise therapy options in future.

4.6   Resulting Alarm System

We identified the "bpt" system as a performant classifier (considering the time period L3). In fact, our aim is not to predict the patients' outcome within the last three days of their ICU stay. We want to warn the physician *during* the *entire* ICU stay if a patient is critical. To set up the alarm system we proceed as follows: We tried out different output thresholds for our neuro-fuzzy system, i.e. thresholds for adjusting sensitivity/specifity considering all samples from the time series of the patients. For every sample we generate the alarm "very critical" – using the trained neuro-fuzzy system – if the (normed) output o_d for the class "deceased" is $\geq \kappa_1$ resp. the alarm "critical" if the (normed) output o_d for the class "deceased" is $\kappa_1 > o_d \geq \kappa_2$ with chosen thresholds $\kappa_1 > \kappa_2$. If o_d is $< \kappa_2$ no alarm is given. In this manner we use our outcome predictor, trained within the period L3, as an alarm system for the entire ICU stay. Every time a patient becomes as critical as most of the deceased patients in the last three days, the system generates an alarm.

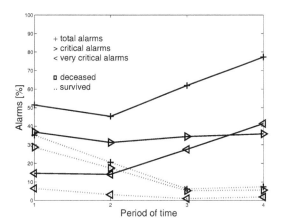

Figure 4. Progression of alarms over time. Critical, very critical and total alarms for deceased and survived patients. Mean values over test patients. Periods: $1 =$ first three days (F3), $2 =$ first half of ICU stay, $3 =$ second half of ICU stay, $4 =$ last three days (L3).

In Fig. 4 we present the average percentage of alarms given for the patients for different time periods. Ten times more alarms in the last three days for deceased patients than for survived patients seems to be reliable for a bedside system.

5   Conclusion

Our aim was the extraction of information from septic shock patient measurement data. For this purpose we applied an efficient improved neuro-fuzzy algorithm to generate rules. We obtained interesting rules for the classes of deceased and survived patients. A detailed comparison of the classification performance of scores showed that the best score for septic shock outcome diagnosis is the SOFA score. We identified the systolic and diastolic blood pressure/thrombocytes ("bpt") system as the most relevant for outcome prediction. It is possible to achieve a similar classification performance as by the SOFA score, but with less variables (3 instead of 10) together with a rule-based explanation.

Our alarm system produces reliable alarms (in the last three days of the ICU stay ten times more alarms for deceased patients then for survivors). Finally, in April 2002 we started a multicenter study to check the clinical usefulness of our system.

Acknowledgement: Our work is supported by the German Research Foundation (DFG). The authors thank all the participants of the MEDAN working group.

References

1. Hanisch, E., Encke, A.: Intensive Care Management in Abdominal Surgical Patients with Septic Complications, published in: E. Faist (ed.) Immunological Screening and Immunotherapy in Critically Ill Patients with Abdominal Infections. Springer-Verlag (2001) 71–138
2. Vanderschueren, S. et al.: Thrombocytopenia and Prognosis in Intensive Care. Crit. Care Med. **28** (2000) 1871–1876
3. Paetz, J., Hamker, F., Thöne, S.: About the Analysis of Septic Shock Patient Data. 1st Int. Symp. on Medical Data Analysis. LNCS Vol. 1933. Springer-Verlag (2000) 130–137
4. Huber, K.-P., Berthold, M.R.: Building Precise Classifiers With Automatic Rule Extraction. Proc. of the IEEE Int. Conf. on Neural Networks **3** (1995) 1263–1268
5. Paetz, J.: Metric Rule Generation with Septic Shock Patient Data. Proc. of the 1st IEEE Int. Conf. on Data Mining (2001) 637–638
6. Brause, R., Hamker, F., Paetz, J.: Septic Shock Diagnosis by Neural Networks and Rule Based Systems. In: M. Schmitt et al. (eds.) Computational Intelligence Processing in Medical Diagnosis. Physica-Verlag (2002) 323–356
7. Vincent, J.-L. et al.: The SOFA (Sepsis-Related Organ Failure Assessment) Score to Describe Organ Dysfunction/Failure. Intensive Care Med. **22** (1996) 707–710
8. Knaus, W.A. et al.: APACHE II: A Severity of Disease Classification System. Crit. Care Med. **13**(10) (1985) 818–829
9. Le Gall, J.R. et al.: A New Simplified Acute Physiology Score (SAPS II) Based on a European / North American Multicenter Study. The Journ. of the Am. Med. Assoc. **270** (1993) 2957–2963
10. Marshall, J.C. et al.: Multiple Organ Dysfunction Score: A Reliable Descriptor of a Complex Clinical Outcome. Crit. Care Med. **23**(10) (1995) 1638–1652

Appendix A – The Neuro-fuzzy Algorithm

parameters: p_i^s (i-th neuron of class s), w_i^s (weight of p_i^s)

1. reset weights:
for s = 1 **to** number of classes **do**
   for i = 1 **to** m_s (number of neurons for class s) **do**
      $w_i^s := 0$;
      set core rule volume of p_i^s to zero;
   end
end

2. consider all samples $(x; c)$ with c as class label of x:
for all samples x **do**
   if p_i^c covers x **then**

3.   cover:
       $w_i^c := w_i^c + 1$;
       adjust core region, so that it covers x;

4. commit new neuron:
   else
       $z_{m_c+1}^c := x$;
       set core rule volume of $p_{m_c+1}^c$ to zero;
       set support rule volume to infinity;

5.   **for** $s \neq c$, $1 \leq j \leq m_s$ **do**
       shrink $p_{m_c+1}^c$ using z_j^s;
    end
    $m_c := m_c + 1$;
    $w_{m_c}^c := 1$;
   end

6. shrink conflict neurons:
   for $s \neq c$, $1 \leq j \leq m_s$ **do**
       shrink p_j^s using x;
   end
end

Appendix B – The Datasets

We use the following abbreviations: CVP = central venous pressure, PTT = partial thromboplastin time, TPT = thromboplastin time, AT = anti throm- bin, EK = erythrocytes concentrate, FFP = fresh frozen plasma, I:E = inspi- ratory:expiratory (pressure). The units in the following datasets are only men- tioned once:

frequent16: heart frequency [1/min], systolic blood pressure [mmHg], diastolic blood pressure [mmHg], temperature [°C], CVP [mmHg], O_2 saturation [%], leukocytes [1000/μl], haemoglobin [g/dl], haematocrit [%], thrombocytes [1000/ μl], PTT [s], sodium [mmol/l], potassium [mmol/l], creatinin [mg/dl], blood sugar [mg/dl], urine volume [ml].

haemogram: leukocytes, erythrocytes [1000/μl], thrombocytes, TPT [%], PTT [s], haemoglobin, haematocrit, thrombin time [s], AT3 [%], fibrinogen [mg/dl], total protein [g/dl], blood sugar [mg/dl], EK [ml], FFP [ml].

heart: heart frequency, systolic blood pressure, diastolic blood pressure, CVP, cristalloids [ml], colloids [ml], adrenaline [μg/kg/min], noradrenaline [μg/kg/min], dopamine [μg/kg/min], dobutamine [μg/kg/min].

lungs: arterial pO_2 [mmHg], arterial pCO_2 [mmHg], base excess [-], bicarbonat [mmol], O_2 saturation, O_2 medication [l/min], Peak [cmH_2O], I:E [-], respiratory frequency [1/min], FiO_2 [%], PEEP [mmHg].

bac: FiO_2, PEAK, respiratory frequency, adrenaline, noradrenaline, dopamine, dobutamine.

Determination of Functional Relationships for Continuous Variables by Using a Multivariable Fractional Polynomial Approach

Dr. Willi Sauerbrei[1] and Prof. Dr. Patrick Royston[2]

[1]Institut für Medizinische Biometrie und Medizinische Informatik, Universitätsklinikum Freiburg, Stefan-Meier-Strasse 26, D- 79104 Freiburg
[2] MRC Clinical Trials Unit, London, UK

Abstract. Determination of a transformation which better describes the functional relationship between the outcome and a continuous covariate may substantially improve the fit of a model. The so-called fractional polynomials approach was proposed to investigate in a systematic fashion possible improvements in fit by the use of non-linear functions. The approach may be used to combine variable selection with the determination of functional relationships for continuous regressors in a multivariable setting, and is applicable to a wide range of general regression models. We will demonstrate some advantages of this flexible family of parametric models by discussing several aspects of modelling the continuous risk factors in a large cohort study. We will also use data halving and the bootstrap to investigate whether the considerable flexibility of the fractional polynomials approach causes instability in the selected functions.

1. Introduction

In epidemiological and clinical studies data on many variable are almost always recorded. The aim is to investigate them simultaneously and to identify those which have an influence on the outcome of interest. One central issue centers around variable selection procedures, but that topic will not be considered here. A recommendable monograph is by Miller (1990). Some approaches to tackle problems caused by these procedures are discussed in Sauerbrei (1999). In combination with variable selection it is also important to deal with non-linearity in the relationship between the outcome variable and a continuous or ordered predictor. Traditionally, such predictors are entered into stepwise selection procedures as linear terms or as dummy variables obtained after grouping. The assumption of linearity may be incorrect, leading to a mis-specified final model in which a relevant variable may not be included (e.g. because the true relationship with the outcome is non-monotonic) or in which the assumed functional form differs substantially from the unknown true form. Categorization introduces problems of defining cut-points (Altman et al. 1994), over-parameterization and loss of efficiency (Lagakos, 1988). In any case a cut-point model is an unrealistic way to describe a relationship between a predictor and an

A. Colosimo et al. (Eds.): ISMDA 2002, LNCS 2526, pp. 53-60, 2002.

outcome variable because it is unreasonable to postulate that risk suddenly increases as a category cut-point is crossed. Also, the results depend on the number and choice of cut-points. An alternative approach is to keep the variable continuous and to allow some form of non-linearity. A flexible family of parametric models is based on so-called fractional polynomial (FP) functions (Royston and Altman (1994)). Here, one, two or more terms of the form X^p are fitted, the exponents p being chosen from a small preselected set of integer and non-integer values. FP functions encompass conventional polynomials as a special case. For the analysis of a large cohort-study we will use an algorithm based on fractional polynomials to combine variable selection with determination of functional relationships for several continuous predictors simultaneously (Sauerbrei and Royston (1999)). To illustrate issues of stability in a simple fashion, we will repeat the selection procedure in two halves of the data defined by a single random 50:50 split. Furthermore this issue will be investigated by a small bootstrap study.

2. Fractional Polynomial Approach

Suppose that we have an outcome variable which is related to a single continuous or ordered-categorical factor x. The natural starting point, the straight line model b_0+b_1x is often adequate, but other models must be investigated for possible improvements in fit. We look for non-linearity by fitting a first-order fractional polynomial (FP-1) to the data. The best power transformation x^p is found, with the power p chosen from the set of candidates $\{-2, -1, -0.5, 0, 0.5, 1, 2, 3\}$, where x^0 denotes log x. For example, for p=-2 the model is b_0+b_1/x^2. The set includes the straight line (i.e. no transformation, p=1), and the reciprocal, logarithmic, square root and square transformations. A test for the need for an FP-1 transformation is performed by comparing the difference in model deviances with a χ^2 distribution on 1 degree of freedom.

Whether or not goodness-of-fit tests show that a first-degree fractional polynomial provides an unsatisfactory fit to the data, it is worth considering second-degree fractional polynomials (FP-2), which offer considerably more flexibility. In particular, many functions with a single turning point (a minimum or a maximum), including some so called J-shaped relationships, can be accommodated. For example, Figure 1 shows four curves with first power −2 and different second powers. The present curves demonstrate some of the shapes that are possible; for further details see Royston and Altman (1994). The models are of the form $b_0+b_1x^p+b_2x^q$ or, for the mathematical limit p=q, $b_0+b_1x^p+b_2x^p$ log x. As before, p and q are chosen from among the set $\{-2, -1, 0, -0.5, 0, 0.5, 1, 2, 3\}$. The best fit among the 36 combinations of such powers is defined as that which maximizes the likelihood. A first-degree model is nested within a second-degree one so that the deviance of the latter is guaranteed to be smaller. Strategies to select the preferred function based on model deviances are proposed by Royston and Altman (1994) with some modifications by Sauerbrei and Royston (1999). The latter paper concentrates on the situation of several predictors and considers the issue of how to incorporate medical knowledge (e.g. function has to be monotonic). This multivariable FP (M-FP) procedure combines backward elimination with an algorithm which is analogous to backfitting to select the best FP transformation for each predictor with the transformations of the other predictors temporarily held fixed.

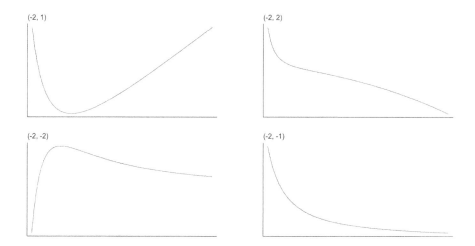

Fig. 1. Four FP curves with first power −2 and different second powers

To demonstrate the importance of investigating non-linearity we give the estimated functional influence of age on the log relative risk of recurrence or death for patients with breast cancer by three approaches (Figure 2). Assuming a linear function, age is not a significant predictor; the function plotted is nearly parallel with the x-axis because the slope parameter is very close to zero. With a step-function approach age is also not significant. Because of the well-known problem of the optimal cut-point approach the cut-points were specified data-independently before the analysis. The M-FP approach exhibited a highly significant influence of an FP-2 function with powers (-2, -0.5). More details may be found in Sauerbrei et al (1999). Flexible modelling of continuous functions, especially when combined with variable selection in a multivariable model, may cause instability (excessive variability and/or artefactual features) in the functions selected. Royston and Sauerbrei (2002) considered how to assess possible instability in multivariable fractional polynomial models by using bootstrap resampling. In each bootstrap replicate they applied the algorithm for simultaneous selection of variables and selection of functions for continuous predictors. They investigated dependencies among inclusion fractions and simplified versions of the functions for each predictor. Clearly, inclusion or exclusion of a correlated predictor may have a substantial influence on the function selected. By a detailed investigation in the framework of log-linear models, they were able to define reasonably large subsets of bootstrap replications in which the functional form of the predictors was similar to the function proposed from the original analysis. They concluded from this bootstrap investigation that their multivariable selection algorithm can find stable models despite the considerable flexibility of the FP family.

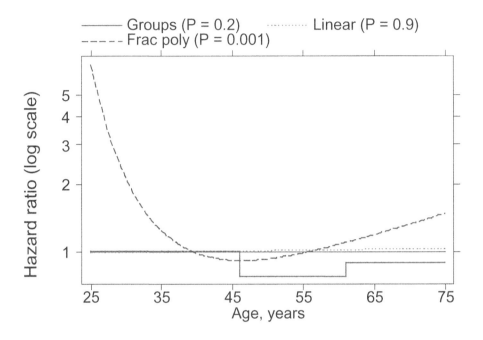

Fig. 2. Estimated functional influence of age for patients with breast cancer by three approaches

3. M-FP Analysis of the Whitehall I Cohort Study

Whitehall I is a prospective, cross-sectional cohort study of 18403 male British Civil Servants employed in London (Marmot et al (1984)). Its aim was to examine factors which influence all-cause and disease-specific death rates in a defined population. At entry to the study, each participant provided demographic details, filled in a health questionnaire and gave a blood sample for biochemical analysis. For present purposes we focus on the data with complete 10-year follow-up (N = 17260, 1670 deaths from any cause). We consider age, cigarette smoking, systolic blood pressure and cholesterol as continuous risk factors for all-cause mortality, adjusting for Civil Service job grade (4 categories) as confounder. The response variable is binary, death within the 10-year follow-up period. The model estimates the log odds of dying as a function of the risk factors interest. For more details see Royston et al (1999).

Results of the M-FP approach are summarized in Tab 1 and graphically presented in Figure 3. For reasons of biological plausibility we allowed only monotone (i.e. FP-1) functions to be selected for cigarette smoking. Age and cholesterol seem to be linearly related to the outcome. For cigarette smoking the transformation $x^{0.5}$ was selected. For systolic blood pressure a FP-2 function fitted the data substantially better (p=0.003) than the best FP-1 transformation.

Part	Age	Cigarettes*	Cholesterol	Systolic-BP
All data	Linear	0.5	Linear	-2, -2
Half 1	Linear	0.5	Linear	3
Half 2	-2	Log	Linear	3

* for biological plausibility, only monotone (FP-1) functions allowed

Table 1. Influence of four continuous variables on 10 year mortality rate in Whitehall I. Selected functions with the M-FP approach in all data and in the two sets from data halving. All models are adjusted for job grade (3 binary dummies).

As shown in Figure 3, postulated functions in the two halves of the data were similar with the main exception of small values for systolic blood pressure. In both halves of the data the test favoring an FP-2 over an FP-1 function just failed significance (p-values 0.055 and 0.062), which may simply be caused by the reduced power because of the smaller sample size. In Figure 4b we show the best FP-2 functions in both halves, clearly demonstrating the similarity in all three postulated functions. A further difference can be seen for the age function which is slightly non-linear in one half of the data; however this is restricted to the small subgroup of men younger than 45 years. Here some instability is present as there are only 26 deaths in this subset.

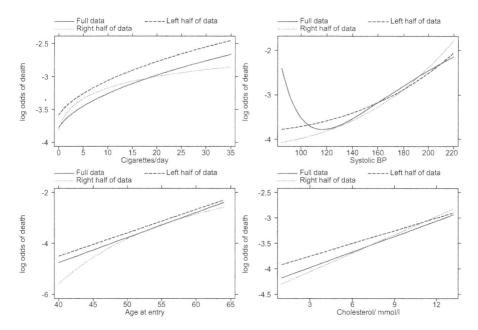

Fig. 3. Selected functions for all four predictors on all data and the two random halves.

A more detailed analysis of the stability of functions selected by using the bootstrap was proposed by Royston and Sauerbrei (2002). The algorithm is applied within each replication to select a final model. The main emphasis is the investigation of the dependencies among inclusion fractions for each predictor and the simplified versions of the functions selected. The M-FP algorithm was applied in each of 100 bootstrap replications to select variables and functions within the Whitehall 1 dataset. All the continuous predictors were selected in all replications except for cholesterol, which was selected in 96. For cigarettes, age and cholesterol, an FP-1 function was always selected, whereas for blood pressure, an FP-2 function was chosen in 89% of replications. In this example dependencies among inclusion fractions seem to be less important.

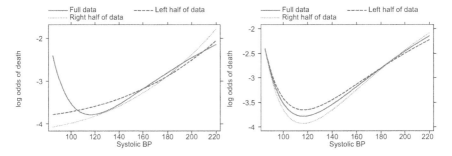

Fig. 4. Selected functions for systolic blood pressure. Selected from M-FP (left), best FP-functions in the two halves of the data (right).

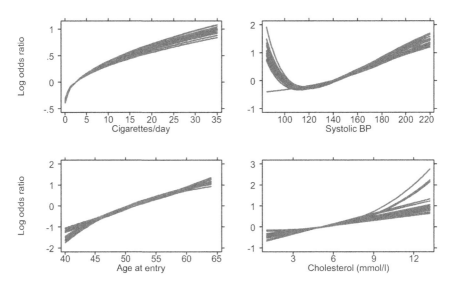

Fig. 5. Sets of 20 fitted curves for each of the four continuous covariates in the Whitehall 1 cohort study. Each curve is standardized to have mean zero and was estimated from a bootstrap sample by applying the M-FP algorithm with function and variable selection.

In Figure 5 we show the fitted functions for the 4 continuous predictors, estimated within each of 20 bootstrap replications chosen at random from the 100. It is clear that the functions estimated for a given predictor are similar in form and appear stable. The function for systolic blood pressure is usually unimodal, but as reported above, in a few cases an FP-1 function is selected, leading to a monotone function. This instability is also seen in Figure 4, where the sample size has been reduced by 50%. It suggests that despite the large sample size, there is not quite enough information in the data to resolve beyond doubt the shape of the mortality function for persons with low blood pressure. Some instability is seen also in the cholesterol function for high values, where the level of risk appears not to be accurately estimated.

Based on the experiences of Royston and Sauerbrei (2002), we expect that stability may be slightly increased by defining sensible subsets of bootstrap replications in which the correlation structure of the other variables selected is allowed for. However, such an investigation is beyond the scope of this paper.

Discussion

Based on an example from the literature and new analyses of a large cohort study, we have shown the importance of determining the functional relationships for continuous variables. Using the multivariable fractional polynomial approach, we showed that non-linear functions fitted the data significantly better for two of the four continuous variables. In this paper there is insufficient space available to consider any of the competitors proposed in the literature (e.g. splines or kernel methods).

However, we feel that fractional polynomials offer the best compromise with respect to important issues such as fitting of the data, simplicity for presentation and practical use, and stability of the function chosen. These issues are discussed in detail in some of the references. The investigation with data halving demonstrated for systolic blood pressure that a 'better' function may be missed because of lack of power for our test-based approach. We speculate that in many analyses in the literature a linear relationship is wrongly postulated because non-linear functions were never considered or because the sample size was too low to give convincing evidence in favour of a non-linear function. We tried to demonstrate with our small bootstrap investigation that the multivariable FP-algorithm can produce models which are fairly stable. So far we are not aware of any detailed investigation of the stability of alternatives to our approach, eg. spline functions to model continuous predictors in a generalized additive model (Hastie and Tibshirani 1990). These functions are more influenced by local features of the data. In the literature they are sometimes used because of their flexibility, but the price for this flexibility may be over-fitting the data and the postulation of curves which may be difficult to interpret and to transfer to other settings.

Our bootstrap investigation may also be considered as a first step towards including model uncertainty in the development process of the function proposed. For a long time it was emphasized that data-dependent modeling may result in over-confident statements about parameter estimates. Several approaches have been proposed in recent years which try to improve the accuracy of predictors and their estimated variance by including model uncertainty in a systematic manner. Most of them use a Bayesian approach (Hoeting et al 1999). An alternative is to use weighted averaging of results from bootstrap replications (Buckland et al (1997)). For our issue of estimating the functional relationship for a continuous variable, the 36 FP-2 functions could be defined as the class of models under consideration. In this context incorporation of model uncertainty would be a special case of the proposal by Augustin et al (2002).

Acknowledgments

We are most grateful to Michael Marmot and Martin Shipley for making the data from the Whitehall I study available to us for analysis.

References

1. Altman DG, Lausen B, Sauerbrei W, Schumacher M: The dangers of using 'optimal' cutpoints in the evaluation of prognostic factors. Journal of the National Cancer Institute, 1994; 86:829-874.
2. Augustin NH, Sauerbrei W, Schumacher M: Incorporating model selection uncertainty into prognostic factor model predictions. Freiburg Centre for Data Analysis and Modelling, No. 76, 2002
3. Buckland S, Burnham KP, Augustin NH: Model selection: an integral part of inference. Biometrics, 1997; 53:603-618
4. Hastie TJ, Tibshirani, RJ: Generalized Additive Models, 1990; New York: Chapman and Hall
5. Hoeting JA, Madigan D, Raftery AE, Volinsky CT: Bayesian model averaging:a tutorial (with discussion). Statistical Science, 1999; 14:382-417
6. Marmot MG, Shipley MJ, Rose G: Inequalities in death – specific explanations of a general pattern? Lancet, 1984; i:1003-1006.
7. Miller AJ: Subset selection in regression, 1990; New York: Chapman and Hall
8. Lagakos SW: Effects of mismodelling and mismeasuring explanatory variables on tests of their association with a response variable. Statistics in Medicine, 1988; 14: 1999-2008.
9. Royston P, Altman DG: Regression using fractional polynomials of continuous covariates: parsimonious parametric modeling (with discussion). Applied Statistics, 1994; 43: 429-467.
10. Royston P, Ambler G, Sauerbrei W: The use of fractional polynomials to model continuous risk variables in epidemiology. International Journal of Epidemiology, 1999; 28:964-974
11. Royston P, Sauerbrei W: Stability of multivariable fractional polynomial models with selection of variables and transformations: a bootstrap investigation. Statistics in Medicine, 2002, to appear
12. Sauerbrei W: The use of resampling methods to simplify regression models in medical statistics. Applied Statistics, 1999; 48:313-329.
13. Sauerbrei W, Royston P: Building multivariable prognostic and diagnostic models: transformation of the predictors using fractional polynomials. Journal of the Royal Statistic Society, 1999; 162: 71-94.
14. Sauerbrei W, Royston P, Bojar H, Schmoor C, Schumacher M for the German Breast Cancer Study Group (GBSG): Modeling the effects of standard prognostic factors in node-positive breast cancer. British Journal of Cancer, 1999; 79: 1752-1760.

Nonlinear Oscillation Models for Spike Separation

Tetyana I. Aksenova[1,4], Olga K. Chibirova[1,4],
Alim-Louis Benabid[1,2], Alessandro E.P. Villa[1,2,3]

1 - Laboratory of Preclinical Neuroscience, INSERM U 318, CHU Michallon, Pav. B,
BP 217, 38043 Grenoble Cedex 9, France
Tatyana.Aksyonova@ujf-grenoble.fr
2 - Laboratoire de Neurobiophysique, Université Joseph Fourier - Grenoble 1, CHU Michallon,
Pav. B, BP 217, 38043 Grenoble Cedex 9, France
3 - Laboratoire de Neuroheuristique, Institut de Physiologie, Université de Lausanne,
7 Rue du Bugnon, 1005 Lausanne, Switzerland
4 – Laboratory of Nonlinear Analysis, Institute of Applied System Analysis,
Pr. Peremogy 37, Kiev, Ukraine

Abstract. The present study reports an approach for automatic classification of extracellularly recorded action potentials (spikes). The recorded signal is observed at discrete times and characterized by high level of background noise and occurrence of the spikes at random time. The classification of spike waveform is considered as a pattern recognition problem of special segments of signal that correspond to the appearance of spikes. The spikes generated by one neuron should be recognized as members of the same class. We describe the spike waveform as an ordinary differential equation with perturbation. This allows us to characterize the signal distortions in both amplitude and phase. We have developed an iteration-learning algorithm that estimates the number of classes and their centers according to the distance between spike trajectories in phase space. The estimation of trajectories in phase space required calculation of the first and second order derivatives and the integral operators with piecewise polynomial kernels were used. This approach is computational efficient and of potential use for real time situations, in particular during neurosurgical procedures.

Introduction

The success of deep brain stimulation techniques for treatment of motor disorders (in particular Parkinson's Disease) opens new perspectives to the development of electrophysiological techniques in contemporary neurosurgery [1,2]. The recording of extracellular neuronal activity during the neurosurgical operation represents a crucial step because it provides unique information about the pattern of neuronal activity of the regions explored during the electrode penetrations. However, the quality of the information gained during the advancement of the electrode depends on the separation from the background noise of few action potentials (spikes) from the same electrode. Several spike sorting techniques have been developed in recent years [3].

A. Colosimo et al. (Eds.): ISMDA 2002, LNCS 2526, pp. 61-70, 2002.

It have been determined by the availability of fast computers at cheap price and include computationally intensive methods such as neural networks [4,5] and wavelet transforms [6,7].

Most techniques allow the classification of the signal in the time domain, but can account only for the additive noise. In this article we present a new method of spike sorting based on nonlinear oscillation models, which is potentially able to overcome several limitations of current techniques.

Mathematical Statement of the Problem and General Description of the Model

We suppose that a microelectrode signal $\widetilde{x}(t) = x(t) + \xi(t)$ is observed at discrete times $t=0,1,....$ Here $\xi(t)$ is a sequence of independent identically distributed random variables with zero mean and finite variance ($\sigma_\xi^2 < \infty$). The signal $x(t)$ is characterized by the occurrence of repeated intervals with amplitudes significantly exceeding the variance of $\xi(t)$. These intervals are assumed to correspond to the occurrence of neuronal discharges, i.e. the spikes (Fig. 1).

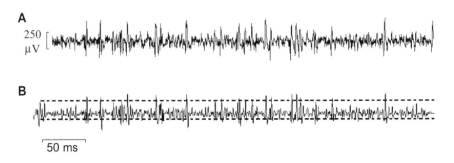

Fig. 1. Example of brain activity observed in the internal segment of the globus pallidus during neurosurgery of dystonia (A) and its derivative (B) with detected spikes. The dashed line corresponds to the threshold.

The spikes $x^i(t_i^*+t)$, $0 < t \leq T^i$ appear at random times t_i^* and have the duration T^i. Otherwise the signal $x(t)$, without noise, equals zero all the time. Each spike is assumed to correspond to the occurrence of a neuronal discharge generated by one among p neurons under observation. Let us denote X_j, $0 \leq j \leq p$ the general population of spikes generated by a single neuron, Let us set the time of spike appearance at zero, thus the general population of spikes generated by a single unit j is denoted as follows, $X_j=\{x^i(t), 0 < t \leq T^i\}_I$. Each general population of spikes corresponds to intervals of the signal with similar waveform. Let us assume that the spikes $x^i(t)$, $0 < t \leq T^i$ from general population X_j are a solution of the same ordinary differential equation with perturbation

$$\frac{d^n x}{dt^n} = f^j\left(x, \ldots, \frac{d^{n-1} x}{dt^{n-1}}\right) + F(x, \ldots, t), \tag{1}$$

where n is the order of the equation, $F()$ is a perturbation function and equation

$$\frac{d^n x}{dt^n} = f^j\left(x, \ldots, \frac{d^{n-1} x}{dt^{n-1}}\right), \tag{2}$$

describes a self-oscillating system with stable limit cycle $\mathbf{x}_j^0(t) = \left(x_1^0(t), \ldots, x_n^0(t)\right)'$ in phase space with co-ordinates $x_1 = x,\; x_2 = \dfrac{dx}{dt}$ ——— for each j, $0 \le j \le p$. T is the period of stable oscillations. The perturbation function $F(x, \ldots, t)$, bounded by a small value, is a random process with zero mean and small correlation time $\tau^* \ll T$.

The mathematical model introduced in (1) and (2) rests on two critical assumptions: (i) the spikes are described by a solution of differential equations with presence of noise in the dynamic equation; (ii) the spikes generated by the same neuron are assumed to be described by the same equation. A successful data analysis can be achieved only if we firstly detect the occurrence of a spike and, secondly, the detected spike should be correctly classified according to the dynamic equation.

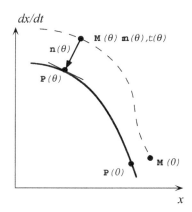

Fig. 2. New variables, i.e. θ and $\mathbf{n}(\theta)$, are introduced to describe the trajectories of the analyzed signal in the phase space. The thick line is the limit trajectory. The length of the vector $|\mathbf{n}(\theta)|$ corresponds to minimal distance between the signal and the limit trajectory.

It is well known [8], that the trajectory of the signal continuously tends to the limit cycle whenever it is found in the neighborhood. The perturbation function $F()$ in (1) tends to displace the trajectories of the signal out from the limit cycle. However, if the perturbation is small enough the trajectories stay in the neighborhood, i.e., the solutions of (1) are similar to one another but they never coincide.

Following [9], we introduce the local coordinates in the neighborhood of the limit cycle. Let us fix an arbitrary point on the limit cycle as a starting point. The position of any arbitrary point P on the limit trajectory can be described by its phase θ, which is a time movement along the limit cycle from a starting point, defined as $P(\theta = 0)$. The phase θ unambiguously characterizes all points of the limit trajectory. Let us assume that f^j in (2) is twice continuously differentiable on all the arguments of the function, thus providing a necessary smoothing. At a point $P(\theta)$ with phase θ it is possible to construct an hyperplane (and only one such hyperplane) that is normal to the limit cycle. Let us consider an arbitrary trajectory of (1) in the neighborhood of limit cycle. Denote $M(\theta)$ the point of its intersection to the hyperplane of phase θ and set the point of phase zero $M(0)$, $\theta = 0$ as the initial point for analyzed trajectory. Any trajectory can be described by variables $\mathbf{n}(\theta)$ and $t(\theta)$ (Fig. 2) where $\mathbf{n}(\theta)$ is a vector of deviation defined by $M(\theta)$ and its orthogonal projection $P(\theta)$ on the limit trajectory. The second variable $t(\theta)$ is a time movement along the trajectory from the initial point $M(0)$ to the analyzed point $M(\theta)$. Thus, the limit trajectory is defined by $\mathbf{n}(\theta) \equiv \mathbf{0}$ and $t(\theta) \equiv \theta$, where $\mathbf{0}$ is a vector with all components equal to 0.

Let us consider phase θ, such as $0 < \theta \leq T$, i.e. runing from 0 to T. For the stable limit cycle the phase equals to the time motion, so that the limit cycle can be described as $\mathbf{x}^0_j(\theta)$. Let us consider the segments of an abitrary signal trajectory $\mathbf{x}^i(t(\theta))$, referred to as a cycles. Each general population X_j of curves is formed by cycles in the neighborhood of a stable limit cycle of the appropriate equation. If the signal corresponds to an extracellular electrophysiological recording, the cycles of the trajectory described by Eq. (1), with $x^i(t)$, $0 < t \leq T^i$, may be interpreted as the waveforms corresponding to the neuronal discharges where T^i is the duration of the spike. The limit trajectory $\mathbf{x}_j^0(t)$, $0 < t \leq T$ corresponds to an ideal spike without noise, referred to as "undisturbed spike". Then the duration T^i of a spike $x^i(t)$ can be written as a function of the period of the stable oscillations $T^i = t^i(T)$.

Our goal is to develop a real-time algorithm for spike recognition according to the dynamic equation (1) in the case when the number of neurons is unknown.

The method presented in this paper includes several steps. At first, the problem of spike classification is reduced to the separation of a mixture of normal distributions in a transformed feature space. Secondly, the estimation of the trajectories in the phase space must be calculated, by the appropriate numerical algorithms. Thirdly, a procedure for detecting a spike occurrence out of the noisy signal must be performed.

Feature Space Transformation

The problem of spike sorting according to self oscillating models with perturbations, i.e. (1) and (2), is reduced to the separation of a mixture of normal distributions in the transformed feature space where the undisturbed spikes $x_j^0(t)$, $0 < t \leq T$, where T is the duration of spike, determine the centers of the classes X_j. Vectors $\mathbf{n}_i(\theta)$ are characterized by an asymptotically Gaussian distribution for any θ in case of uncorrelated noise $F()$. The mean trajectory of signals in phase space converges to the limit cycle in linear approximation if the number of averaged trajectories increases infinitely. Thus, the mean trajectory represents an unbiased estimation of the limit cycle in the first approximation: $n^*(\theta) \approx 0$, $t^*(\theta) \approx 0$ [9]. These properties allow us to estimate the limit cycle by calculating the mean trajectory of the signal in the phase space and then to estimate an "undisturbed spike" (an ideal spike in phase space) that can be used as a template for spike sorting.

Let us refer to the space $\mathbf{R}^T$ of features $x(t_i)$, $t_i = 1, ..., T$ as a standard feature space with dimension T. Let us consider the space $\mathbf{R}^{n \times T}$, with dimension $n \times T$, of features

$$(\mathbf{x}(t(\theta_1))' \mid \mathbf{x}(t(\theta_2))' \mid \ ... \ \mid \mathbf{x}(t(\theta_T))')', \ \mathbf{x}(t(\theta_i)) = \left(x_1(t(\theta_i)), ..., x_n(t(\theta_i)) \right)', \text{ where}$$

$x_1 = x$, $x_2 = \dfrac{dx}{dt}$ ———. It is important to note that the partition of

the interval of spike observation becomes generally irregular in time, i.e. $t(\theta_{i+1}) - t(\theta_i) \neq 1$. Let us consider a new feature space Ω, with features $\mathbf{x}(t(\theta_i))$, $1 = \theta_1 < ... < \theta_T = T$, $\Delta\theta = 1$, with the Euclidean norm as

$$\|\mathbf{x}\|_\Omega = \left(\sum_{\theta_i} \sum_{0 \le j \le n-1} \left(\frac{d^j x}{dt^j}(t(\theta)) \right)^2 \right)^{1/2}$$

The vector $n(\theta) = \mathbf{x}^j(t(\theta_i)) - \mathbf{x}^0(\theta_i)$ has an asymptotically normal distribution with mathematical expectation close to zero for each class X_j. In the new feature space Ω we have obtained p normal distributed classes and the undisturbed spike $\mathbf{x}_j^0$ corresponds to the center of class X_j.

Estimation of the Trajectory in the Phase Space

Our method requires the estimation of the signal trajectory in phase space. Higher-order derivatives of the signal should be calculated in presence of noise that seriously affects the calculations. In recent studies [10,11], we proposed to describe the signal trajectory in phase space using coordinates $D_\alpha^0 x$, $D_\alpha^1 x$, ..., $D_\alpha^{n-1} x$ instead of origi-

nal $x, \dfrac{dx}{dt}, \cdots, \dfrac{d^{n-1} x}{dt^{n-1}}$, where D_α^k are integral operators

$$D_\alpha^k x(t) = \int_R \omega_\alpha^k(\tau - t) x(\tau) d\tau$$

and the kernel function ω_α satisfies the following three conditions:
a) $\omega_\alpha(t) = 0$, if $|t| > \alpha$?
b) $\displaystyle\int_R \omega_\alpha(t)dt = 1$;   (3)
c) ω_α has n continuous derivatives.

Any function satisfying the conditions set by Eqs. (3) can be used as a kernel function. The selection of both the kernel function and the value of the parameter α depend on the order of the derivative to be calculated and the level of additive noise. A computationally efficient algorithm of derivative estimation [12] is used to calculate $D_\alpha^k x$.

Spike Detection Procedure

The procedure of detection of neuronal discharges—the spikes—is important to determine the time interval of the signal that corresponds to spike occurrences. The spikes are usually characterized by amplitudes significantly larger than the level of background noise and their occurrence may be detected by threshold crossing. In present study instead of the signal itself we considered the first derivative of the signal for filtering low frequency noise.

Let us consider the observed signal as a mixture of noise $\xi(t)$ and spikes. If the probability of spikes occurrence is small enough, then the parametric values of the mixture are close to the noise itself. Then, the values of the mixture can be used instead of the noise characteristics even if such estimation is biased. The same estimation can be also used for the derivatives since its calculation is reduced to the summa-

tion $D_\alpha^k x(t) = \sum_{-\alpha}^{\alpha} A_i\, x(t)$. For the signal with additive noise $\tilde{x}(t) = x(t) + \xi(t)$ we

have $D_\alpha^k \tilde{x}(t) = D_\alpha^k x(t) + D_\alpha^k \xi(t)$ such   that   the   noise   for   derivative

$D_\alpha^k \xi(t) = \sum_{-\alpha}^{\alpha} A_i\, \xi(t)$ is a random variable with zero mean and variance $\sigma^2_{D\xi} = \sigma^2_{\xi}$

$\sum_{-\alpha}^{\alpha} A_i^2$. We can choose an appropriate level of confidence and find the threshold for

spike detection $\boldsymbol{R}_{detect}$ by considering the distribution of $D_\alpha^1 \xi(t)$ as normal, according to the central limit theorem.

Learning Algorithm for Spike Separation

An unsupervised learning algorithm for spike sorting is necessary in order to provide a fast and easy-to-use selection tool to a user during a real-time experiment or during a human surgical intervention. The unsupervised learning algorithm scans a learning set formed by few tens of spike occurrences, usually corresponding to few minutes of recording time, and estimates the number of classes and their centers by measuring the distances between their trajectories in phase space. The rationale is that in case of a Gaussian distribution the mean corresponds to the maximum of the probability density. In a Gaussian distribution, where E is the mathematical expectation, the value $x^* = Ex$ provides the maximum of $P(|x - x^*| < R)$ for any given parameter R. Then, the mean trajectory is estimated by an iterative procedure that detects the spike with maximal probability density in its neighborhood. This spike may be viewed as a "template" spike representative of its class.

If the aim is to identify only one class of spikes the first step of the iterative procedure consists in the selection of an arbitrary spike x_0 as an initial estimate of the center of the class. Its R-neighborhood $\mathbf{R}_0 = \{x: ||x-x_0||_\Omega < R\}$ is constructed on the learning data set. Then we search for the element x_1 that provides the minimum sum of distances

$$x_1 = \arg\min_{x^* \in R_0} \sum_{x \in R_0} \left\| x^* - x \right\|_\Omega \tag{4}$$

and such element is considered as the next approximation. Then, we construct the R-neighborhood of the spike x_1, $\mathbf{R}_1 = \{x: ||x-x_1||_\Omega < R\}$ and so on. Due to the symmetry and modality properties of the normal distribution this procedure converges to a mean value which does not depend on the choice of the parameter R. However, a larger training set is required for smaller values of R.

For the simultaneous search of several classes let us consider that the maxima of the density of joint distributions are near the centers of the classes if the classes are well separated. Thus, it is sufficient to select the initial estimate points in the neighborhood of each maximum in order to detect all centers of the classes. The initial estimates are calculated iteratively following the next procedure:

Step 1 – the first detected spike is selected as the first initial estimate.

i-step - The distances to all available initial estimates that were chosen at previous *steps* are calculated for the *i*-th spike. If all distances to the analyzed spike are larger than the threshold R, then the spike is appended to the initial estimates.

All chosen initial estimates are used in the iterative procedure of the centers of classes estimation up to its termination. The spikes x_i, see (4), obtained as a result of such learning are considered as candidates to represent the centers of the classes.

The distribution of the distances from the center to all other spikes belonging to a given class can be used to estimate the class radius. After the estimation of the number of classes and their centers, the simple minimal distance procedure can be used for preliminary classification of the spikes from the learning set. The square of the distance of each spike to the center of its class follows a χ^2 distribution, because vectors $n(\theta)$ are normally distributed. Then, the experimental distribution $p(s)$ was approximated by function χ^2 using the experimental values up to the maximum of the probability density function, i.e. S_{max}. The deviation of the experimental distribution from the fitted χ^2 provides an estimate of the level of noise in the experimental data. If the experimental distribution follows χ^2 and R_{sort} is the threshold used for spike recognition, then the tail of distribution, i.e. $\int_{R_{sort}}^{\infty} \chi^2 ds$, corresponds to set of spikes that were unclassified.

The integral $\int_{S_{max}}^{R_{sort}} \varphi(s)ds$ where $\phi(s) = \begin{cases} p(s) - \chi^2, & \text{if } p(s) > \chi^2 \\ 0, & \text{otherwise} \end{cases}$, corresponds to the misclassified spikes (Fig. 3). In practice the radius of each class was chosen to equalize misclassified and unclassified errors but not more then 3σ.

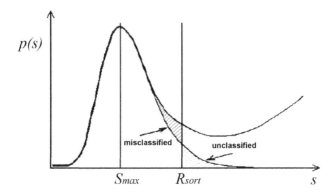

Fig. 3. Experimental distance distribution, the solid line, and chi-square approximation, the dotted line. The vertical lines represent maximum of density probability function, S_{max}, and the threshold used for spike recognition R_{sort}. Area filled with lines corresponds to a misclassification error; the dotted region allows estimating an error of unclassified

After the estimation of the number of classes and their centers the simple minimal distance procedure is used for spike recognition. It corresponds to the construction of piecewise-linear dividing surface in the space Ω.

Model and Method Verification

We used both real and simulated signals of electrophysiological recordings from rat cerebral cortex brain activity for model and method verification. The model of nonlinear oscillation was tested against the hypothesis of normal distribution of the spike amplitudes in the class. The χ^2 test showed that the null hypothesis was accepted with significance level 0.05 for both real and simulated signals. The simulated signal contains three classes of spikes. As a result of learning three classes were found out with 99.9% of correct recognition. To estimate the accuracy of our algorithm in real situation the real electrophysiological signal was superposed to the simulated one. In this case the percentage of correct recognition was 83% for the class with smallest spike amplitude, 92% for the class with middle amplitude and 97% for the class of spikes with largest amplitude. In particular, our method presents an important advantage over methods based on Independent Component Analysis (ICA) and wavelet decomposition because it required little data to perform in a satisfactory way. However we have not carried out a complete comparison between ICA and our own method.

Figure 4 shows an application to a microelectrode recording performed in the human internal segment of the globus pallidus during neurosurgery of dystonia. In this example we show two single units sorted out from the same microelectrode recording and the corresponding autocorrelograms and crosscorrelogram. The average firing rate was 18.3 spikes/s for unit #1 and 13.6 spikes/s for unit #2. The flat crosscorrelogram indicates that there was no sign of synchronization between these units at the time of the recording.

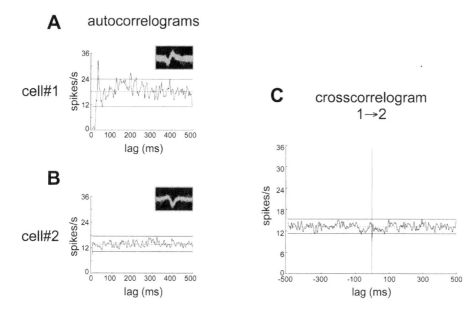

Fig. 4. Microelectrode recording performed in the internal segment of the human globus pallidus during neurosurgery of dystonia. Two spike trains were sorted out simultaneously. The autocorrelograms for the thwo units are shown in (A) and (B). The crosscorrelogram of unit #1 vs. unit #2 is shown in (C). The abscissa full scale is 36 spikes/s and the ordinate is 500 ms. The solid lines correspond to 99% confidence levels assuming Poisson distribution of the point process and the dashed lines correspond to the average.

Conclusion

We have presented a new method for detection and classification of neuronal discharges on the basis of the electrophysiological signal in extracellular recordings. This method will be tested on simulated spikes and will be compared with other approaches used to analyze electrophysiological recordings. We expect that an implementation of our method in the neurosurgical environment will be of extreme interest to assist the neurosurgeons during recordings of human brain activity by deep electrodes. Time is very critical during these operations and a semi-automatic procedure for spike sorting would provide a significant improvement of electrophysiological signal processing over the current procedures. The detected spike patterns could be compared to a library of selected brain structures (such as basal ganglia) established from the results of previous investigations and regularly updated. Patterns of activity obtained from spike train analyses could then be analyzed on-line and provide useful functional hints to the surgeon about the localization of the electrode, through a probabilistic suggested identification of the brain structure being explored.

Acknowledgement

We acknowledge the contribution of Dr. B.A. Wallace and Dr. S. Chabardes for the recording of electrophysiological activiry in the human patients during neurosurgery. This study was partially supported by Swiss NSF 7IP.062620 grant and by Medtronic grant to INSERM U 318. We acknowledge the contribution of Dr. I.V. Tetko and Mr. O.A. Dryga to a preliminary version of this algorithm.

References

1. Krack, P., Pollak, P., Limousin, P., Benazzouz, A., Deuschl, G., Benabid, A.L.: From off-Period Dystonia to Peak-Dose Chorea: the Clinical Spectrum of Varying Subthalamic Nucleus Activity. Brain **122** (1999) 1133-1146
2. Limousin, P., Krack, P., Pollak, P., Benazzouz, A., Ardouin, C., Hoffmann, D., Benabid, A.L.: Electrical Stimulation of the Subthalamic Nucleus in Advanced Parkinson's Disease. New England Journal of Medicine **339(16)** (1998) 1105-1111
3. Schmidt, E.M.: Computer Separation of Multi-Unit Neuroelectric Data: a Review. Journal of Neuroscience Methods **12** (1998) 95-111
4. Chandra, R., Optican, L. M.: Detection, Classification, and Superposition Resolution of Action Potentials in Multiunit Single-Channel Recordings by an On-Line Real-Time Neural Network. IEEE Trans. Biomed. Eng. **44** (1997) 403-412
5. Kim, K.H., Kim, S.J.: Neural Spike Sorting under Nearly 0-dB Signal-to-Noise Ratio Using Nonlinear Energy Operator and Artificial Neural-Network Classifier, IEEE Trans. Biomed. Eng. **47** (2000) 1406-1411
6. Zouridakis, G., Tam, D.C.: Identification of Reliable Spike Templates in Multi-Unit Extracellular Recordings Using Fuzzy Clustering. Computer Methods & Programs in Biomedicine **61** (2000) 91-98
7. Hulata, E., Segev, R., Ben-Jacob, E.: A Method for Spike Sorting and Detection Based on Wavelet Packets and Shannon's Mutual Information, Journal of Neuroscience Methods **117** (2002) 1-12
8. Bogoljubov, N. N., Mitropolsky, Y. A.: Asymptotic Methods in the Theory of non-Linear Oscillations. 2nd edn. Gordon and Breach, New York (1961)
9. Gudzenko, L. I.: Statistical Method for Self-Oscillating System Characteristics Detection. Izvestiia Vuzov Radiophysics **5** (1962) 573-587 (In Russian)
10. Aksenova, T. I., Tetko, I. V., Ivakhnenko, A.G., Villa, A. E. P., Welsh, W. J., Zielinski W. L.: Pharmaceutical Fingerprinting in Phase Space. 1. Construction of Phase Fingerprints. Anal. Chem. **71(13)** (1999) 2423-2430
11. Aksenova, T.I., Tetko, I.V., Dryga, O.A., Chibirova, O.K., Villa, A.E.P.: Detection and Separation of Extracellular Neuronal Discharges. Smart Engineering System Design, Proc. ANNIE'2001, Vol. 11. ASME Press, New York (2001) 557-562
12. Aksenova, T. I., Shelekhova, V. Y.: Fast Algorithms of Derivative Estimation on Noisy Observations. *SAMS* **18-19** (1995) 159-163

Modeling Glucose-Insulin Behavior in Ill Patients (DM Type2)

G. Baratta, F. Barcellona, G. Lucidi, A.M. Bersani

[1]Facoltà di Ingegneria – Università degli Studi "La Sapienza"
Via Eudossiana, 18 – 00184 Rome (Italy)
giubar@inwind.it; f.barcellona@inwind.it; awrluc@vizzavi.it
[2]Dipartimento di Metodi e Modelli Matematici per le Scienze Applicate (Me.Mo.Mat.)
Via A. Scarpa, 16 – 00161 Rome (Italy)
bersani@dmmm.uniroma1.it

Abstract. In this paper we analyze a mathematical model (called MINMOD) that describes the interactions between glucose and insulin in human subjects, in order to realize an adequate model for ill patients, suffering from *Diabetes Mellitus* (DM) Type 2. Our model has been tested on the basis of clinical data and it has correctly reproduced glucose and insulin reply and temporal evolution, according to experimental data test. This model could, in the future, contribute to predict glucose and insulin behavior in ill patients and suggest the adequate treatment.

1. Introduction

Insulin is a protein, made up of 51 amino acids. It is secreted by the pancreas, by means of the so-called "β-cells", in small quantities, which can be highly increased, in order to answer to several inputs (sugars, first of them glucose), amino acids, vagus activity.

It helps glucose and lipids storage in target cells, which are important energy sources. It affects cells growth and the metabolism of many tissues. Besides, it promotes the protein synthesis, increasing the amino acids transport and stimulating ribosome activity. Finally, it helps glycogen synthesis, restoring it after every muscular activity.

It is brought by the bloodstream to specific receptors that have been discovered in quite all the tissues membranes. However, biological effects due to the interaction insulin-receptors have been found in few tissues: liver, muscle, adipose tissue.

Glucose is the most important physiological stimulation for insulin secretion. Insulin reply to a protracted glucose stimulation of the β-cells is split into two phases: a first, high, secretion, rapidly decreasing, and a second, delayed, secretion peak, during all the stimulation period.

A. Colosimo et al. (Eds.): ISMDA 2002, LNCS 2526, pp. 71-78, 2002.

When glucose is no more able to stimulate the β-cells, in the human subject several dysfunctions appear, among which one of the most serious is the so-called "diabetes mellitus" (DM). It is characterized by hyperglycemia, due to a complete absence of insulin or to a partial deficit, related to its reduced biological efficiency. DM can be classified in three forms (see [7]):

a) DM type 1, insulin-dependent (IDMM); it is characterized by a quite complete absence of insulin secretion; it represents the 10-15 % of all the DM pathologies;

b) DM type 2, insulin-independent (NIDMM); it is characterized by a low insulin secretion, associated to tissue refractoriness to insulin activity; it represents the 85-90 % of all the DM pathologies;

c) secondary DM; it includes forms of insulin-refractoriness, connected to other serious diseases, such as muscular dystrophy, myotonic dystrophy etc.

In order to model the mechanism of glucose regulation in the blood, we need to evaluate quantitatively how insulin controls the glucose absorption by the tissues and the stimulation action, done by glucose, on insulin production by the pancreas β-cells.

This information is clinically highly relevant, because it permits to diagnose and classify different pathologies, and consequently to distinguish the forms of glucose intolerance due to DM of type 1 and 2 from secondary DM.

Clinical experience is in general based on experimental tests (IVGTT, IVITT etc.). Unfortunately, these techniques are sometimes not efficient. Consequently the need of satisfactorily mathematical models, able to reproduce insulin-glucose concentrations and temporal behaviors, has recently highly increased.

Several models are presented in classical literature. Already in 1965, Ackerman et al. [1] supplied the first model which studied the interactions between glucose and insulin simultaneously. In early Seventies Grodsky [10] studied models able to explain insulin secretion behavior due to glucose stimulus. The most important result of this study was the description of the multiphase insulin response. Modifying Grodsky's model, Guyton et al. [11] developed a model, on computer, considering some glucose metabolism features, in healthy subjects. The model takes into account heart rate, blood flow, breathing rate etc, and it assumes constant production of fractional insulin, from liver and kidneys.

All this works treat insulin and glucose interaction with highly complexity degrees. Yet, in clinical application, only simple models can find direct utilization. The model which found more interesting applications, in medical practice, is the so called MINMOD by Bergman and Cobelli in the early Eighties. More recently, new interest has been devoted to this topics (see, for example, [2], [5], [6], [9]), trying to improve the original model, for example introducing delays, or suggesting new ones.

We study a MINMOD model, which describes the temporal evolution of insulin and glucose, according to the following compartmental scheme:

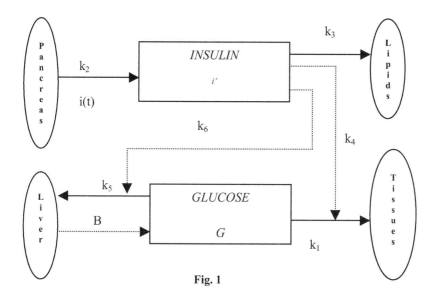

Fig. 1

This model is considered as an optimal model if we require the following assumptions must be fundamental for the simulation of glucose distribution kinetics, following glucose injections:

1) it is sufficient to assume that injected glucose distributes into a single compartment;

2) glucose disappearance occurs in proportion to the plasma glucose concentration;

3) insulin in a compartment remote from plasma (peripheral) accelerates the disappearance of glucose.

The compartments glucose-insulin are represented by functionals, which act on the input functions and whose values are the output functions of the model.

The parameters and variables of the model are the following:

- insulin and glucose concentration in plasma: i' and G; their units are, respectively, $\mu U/ml$ and mg/dl;

- concentration of insulin input: $i(t)$; its unit is $\mu U/ml$;

- glucose concentration in plasma at time 0: B_0; its unit is mg/dl $[minute]^{-1}$;

- concentration of net hepatic glucose: $B = B_0 - (k_5 + k_6\ i')G$; its unit is $mg/dl[minute]^{-1}$;

- kinetics of insulin in the remote compartment: k_2, k_3; their unit is $[minute]^{-1}$;

- effect of glucose to enhance its disappearance: k_1, k_5; their unit is $[minute]^{-1}$;

- effect of remote insulin to enhance glucose disappearance:

k_4, k_6 ; their unit is $ml / \mu U$ $[minute]^{-1}$.

2. The Mathematical Model

In order to analyze the temporal evolution of glucose and insulin, we need to know the temporal variation of the input i(t), described by its kinetic equation; the explicit expression of i(t) is given by i(t) = I(t) – I_b, where I(t) and I_b respectively represent the temporal evolution and the basal value of insulin concentration.

The model considered for the mathematical analysis of the system takes into account the following rearrangements:

$X(t) = (k_4 + k_6) i'(t)$
$p1 = k_1 + k_5$
$p2 = k_3$
$p3 = k_2 (k_4 + k_6)$

The parameters k_i, according to medical experience, can be considered constant.

Thus, the model can be represented by the following system of nonlinear differential equations:

$$\begin{cases} \dfrac{dG}{dt} = -[p_1 + X(t)]G(t) + p_1 G_b & G(0) = G_0 \\[2ex] \dfrac{dX}{dt} = -p_2 X(t) + p_3 [I(t) - I_b] & X(0) = 0 \\[2ex] \dfrac{dI}{dt} = -nI(t) + \gamma[G(t) - h]t & I(0) = I_0 \end{cases}$$

where the first and second equations describe the glucose disappearance, while the third equation rules insulin kinetics.

The estimate of the parameters for a young healthy patient was obtained in [13], by means of a computer routine, based on a modified Marquardt's nonlinear least squares method (see [8], [12]), which uses clinical experimental data, showing the behavior of glucose and insulin during a so-called "frequently-sampled intravenous glucose tolerance" (FSIGT) clinical test, performed in a time interval of 3 hours, which is the optimal one, since in it no significant metabolic variations are observed. The values obtained are the following:

$$p_1 = 0.03082 \quad p_2 = 0.02093 \quad p_3 = 0.00001062 \quad G_0 = 287.0$$
$$n = 0.3 \quad\quad \gamma = 0.003349 \quad\quad h = 89.5 \quad\quad I_0 = 403.4$$

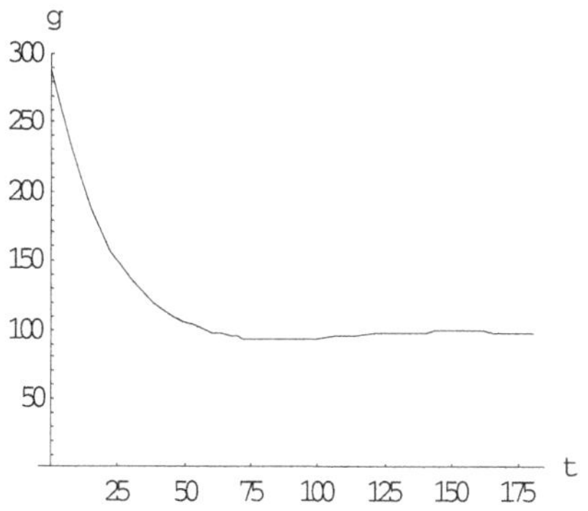

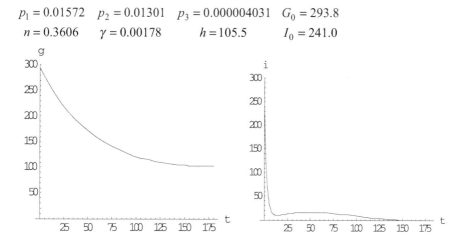

Fig. 2. Temporal evolution of glucose for a young healthy patient.

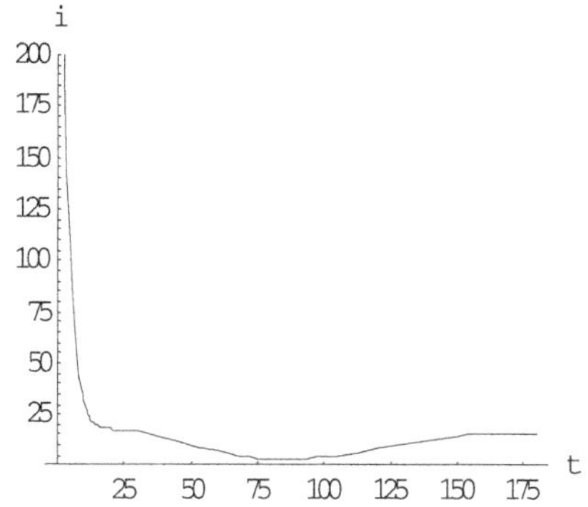

Fig. 3. Temporal evolution of insulin for a young healthy patient.

The parameters estimation for an elderly healthy patient are:

$$p_1 = 0.01572 \quad p_2 = 0.01301 \quad p_3 = 0.000004031 \quad G_0 = 293.8$$
$$n = 0.3606 \quad\quad \gamma = 0.00178 \quad\quad h = 105.5 \quad\quad I_0 = 241.0$$

Fig. 4. Temporal evolution of glucose for an elderly healthy patient.

Fig. 5. Temporal evolution of insulin for an elderly healthy patient.

In both cases, the ingestion of meal at time $t_0 = 0$ implies an initial glucose enhancement, followed by a decreasing phase. Then glucose tends to become stable and later on little oscillations appear around the equilibrium point. Hyperglycemia immediately induces insulin release, followed by a decrease, faster than the corresponding phase in glucose (see, for example, [14]). The slope of the graphs and the duration of the stabilization period depend on the patients' age, as shown in Figs. (2, 3, 4, 5).

3.The Ill Patient

For an ill patient (DM type 2), the differential system must be modified, taking into account partial absence of insulin response and the need of periodic injections of pharmacological agents (e.g. tolbutamide), in order to stimulate insulin receptors, represented by an additive input term, which causes rapid peaks in the graph of insulin temporal evolution, as shown in Figs. (6 and 7). In order to reproduce the experimental data shown in [6], we have translated the injection in mathematical terms by means of a step function with small support, where the height A represents the peak of insulin secretion following the tolbutamide injection (300 mg, see [13]), due to the experimental fact that the tolbutamide injection is approximately constant and short lasting. In [13] the patient receives only one injection, whose duration is taken equal to 1 sec.

$$
\begin{cases}
\dfrac{dG}{dt} = -\left[p_1 + X(t)\right]G(t) + p_1 G_b & G(0) = G_0 \\[2mm]
\dfrac{dX}{dt} = -p_2 X(t) + p_3\left[I(t) - I_b\right] & X(0) = 0 \\[2mm]
\dfrac{dI}{dt} = -nI(t) + \gamma\left[G(t) - h\right]t + A\chi_E(t) & I(0) = I_0
\end{cases}
$$

where E is the set corresponding to the temporal periods during which the injections are performed and χ_E represents the characteristic function of the set E.

Applying the usual least square technique and integrating the differential system gives the following result (the dots are the experimental data, obtained from [13]):

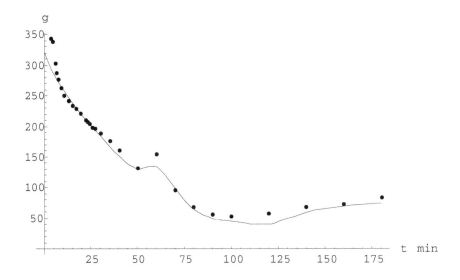

Fig. 6. Temporal evolution of glucose for an ill patient

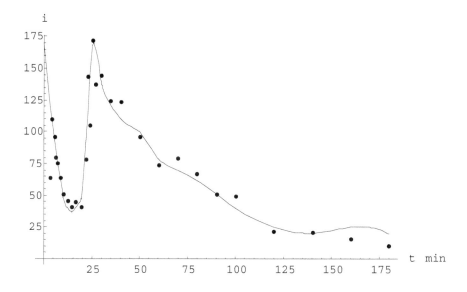

Fig. 7. Temporal evolution of insulin for an ill patient

4. Comments and Further Developments

The model we have analyzed has shown correct insulin responses to glucose variations (in particular peaks) in a young and in an elderly healthy patient, as in an ill one, even if, in the last case, the insulin responses are artificially generated by means of pharmacological agents (e.g. tolbutamide) which stimulate the peripheral tissues insulin receptors, due to their inefficiency caused by DM type 2.

Moreover, since the modified model can reproduce in a sufficiently appropriate way glucose and insulin temporal evolution for an ill patient, suffering from diabetes mellitus type 2, this model could, in the future, if tested with further experimental data, contribute to predict glucose and insulin behavior in ill patients and suggest the adequate treatment.

References

[1] E. Ackerman, L.C. Gatewood, J.W. Rosevear, G.D. Molnar, Model studies of blood-glucose regulation. Bull. Math. Biophys., 27, (1965), pp. 21-37.
[2] G. Baratta, F. Barcellona, G. Lucidi, A.M. Bersani, M. Coli, Stability and equilibrium points in MINMOD for glucose, Proc. VI Congresso Nazionale SIMAI 2002.
[3] R.N. Bergman, C. Cobelli, Minimal modeling, partition analysis and the stimulation of insulin sensitivity. Fed. Proc., 39, (1980), pp. 110-115.
[4] E.R. Carson, C. Cobelli, L. Finkelstein, The mathematical modeling of metabolic and endocrine systems. Wiley & Sons, 1983.

[5] C. Dalla Man, A. Caumo, C. Cobelli, The oral glucose minimal model: estimation of insulin sensitivity from a meal test, IEEE Trans. Biom. Eng., 49, (2002), pp. 419-429.

[6] A. De Gaetano, O. Arino, Mathematical modelling of the intravenous glucose tolerance test, J. Math. Biol., 40, (2000), pp. 136, 168.

[7] G. Faglia, Malattie del sistema endocrino e del metabolismo. McGraw Hill, 1997.

[8] R.A. Fletcher, A modified Marquardt subroutine for non linear least squares, Atomic Energy Research Establishment, Report R AERE-R 6799, 1971.

[9] B. Forzato, Sistemi positivi: modellistica e identificazione della dinamica glucosio-insulina, Tesi di Laurea, Univ. "La Sapienza", Roma (2000).

[10] G.M. Grodsky, A threshold distribution hypothesis for packet storage of insulin and its mathematical modeling, J. Cli. Inv., 51, (1972), pp. 2047, 2059.

[11] J.R. Guyton, O.F. Foster, J.S. Soeldner, M.H. Tan, C.B. Kahn, L. Koncz, R.E. Gleason, A model of glucose-insulin homeostasis in man that incorporates the heterogeneous fast pool theory of pancreatic insulin release, Diabetes, 27, (1978), pp. 1027-1042.

[12] D.W. Marquardt, An algorithm for least squares estimation of non-linear parameters, J. Soc. Ind. Appl. Math., 11 (1963), pp. 431-441.

[13] G. Pacini, R.N. Bergman, MINMOD: a computer program to calculate insulin sensitivity and pancreatic responsivity from the frequently sampled intravenous glucose tolerance test. Computer Methods and Programs in Biomedicine, 23 (1986), pp. 113-122.

[14] G. Van den Berghe et al., Intensive insulin therapy in critically ill patients. N. Engl. J. Med., 345, n. 19 (2001), pp. 1359-1367.

ECG Acquisition and Management System for Knowledge Discovery in Database: Data Modeling, Design, and Implementation

Yongho Cho[1,2], Hosung Kim[1], Myoung-ju Jeon[1], Dongjoo Kang[2]
Hyungsik Choi[3], Jong-min Lee[1], In-young Kim[1], and Sun I. Kim[1]

[1] Biomedical Engineering, Hanyang University, 17 Haengdang-Dong,
Songdong-Gu, Seoul, Korea
{purnima, khs001,jmjsilk}@bme.hanyang.ac.kr
{ljm, iykim, sunkim}@hanyang.ac.kr
[2] Bionet Co., Ltd, #501, KICOX Venture Center, 188-5,
Guro-Dong, Guro-Gu, Seoul, Korea
{purnima, dongjoo}@bme.hanyang.ac.kr
[3] Medical Standard Co., Ltd, HIT, Hanyang University,
17 Haengdang-Dong, Songdong-Gu, Seoul, Korea
hschoi@medicalstandard.com

Abstract. Today, medical science involves large amounts of heterogeneous data, for example biosignals such as Electrocardiograms (ECG), images and other numerical data. Medical images can easily be collected via Picture Archiving and Communication Systems (PACS) and used for Knowledge Discovery in Database (KDD). However, no standard has been defined for the collection and management of ECG, and it is not possible to obtain high quality data in sufficient quantities for KDD. Consequently, it was decided to develop an ECG acquisition and management system. This system is based on five modules constituting an integrated system: ECG equipment, acquisition, archiving, viewer and database. The database model was designed to handle both the ECG examination and patients' records, so that raw ECG's and their associated data, such as weight, age, sex, patients' prescriptions and physicians' analyses, could be simultaneously accessed by KDD. The system developed is able to operate independently or be interfaced with Hospital Information System (HIS).

1 Introduction

The medical field has for many years been fertile ground for the development of new computer and Artificial Intelligence (AI) applications. [1] Large amounts of heterogeneous data have to be managed, for example medical images, biosignals such as ECG's, clinical information such as temperature, cholesterol levels, etc., as well as physicians' interpretations [2], all of which can be used for KDD. Medical images in the field of radiology represent a useful element for KDD, because they almost conform to the Digital Imaging and Communication in Medicine (DICOM) [3] standard and can be collected in large quantities via PACS [4].

However, waveform equipment, including ECG, is not currently compatible with PACS. Also, no standard has yet been defined for the collection and management of

A. Colosimo et al. (Eds.): ISMDA 2002, LNCS 2526, pp. 79–85, 2002.

ECG data. As a result, it is not possible to obtain high quality ECG data in sufficient quantities for KDD. In addition, the presence of certain specific features in ECG's, such as non-standard ECG characteristics, which are absent in non-medical data [5], renders the process of knowledge discovery difficult when it comes to ECG data. Ombrato [3] developed an open system for managing long-term ECG recordings, but it did not consider standards, because the DICOM waveform standard had not been made public in 2000. Its purpose was only to manage ECG data, and so the issue of a database model for KDD was not taken into consideration.

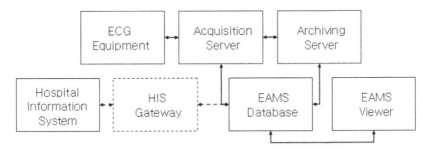

Fig. 1. EAMS Design

In this paper, we propose the ECG Acquisition and Management System (EAMS), which is based on five distinct modules which together constitute an integrated system: ECG equipment, acquisition, archiving, viewer and database. EAMS is based on the DICOM waveform standard. It can therefore be connected with any piece of ECG equipment with only slight modifications, and is suitable for the ECG KDD data repository system. The EAMS database schema is designed and implemented in order to support future ECG KDD systems.

2 System Design

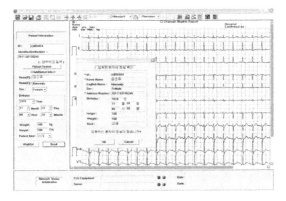

Fig. 2. Acquisition Server

The objective of this research and development is to provide cardiologists with an efficient and convenient ECG examination workflow and the necessary system interface for searching, saving and viewing ECG examination information. In order for physician's to use EAMS with ease, it was designed to resemble PACS, in terms of its design. Both physicians and software engineers participated in the project, in order to maintain coherence between the design architecture and the visual interface. Another goal of this research was to construct a relational model of ECG data and to establish an EAMS database schema for future ECG KDD systems.

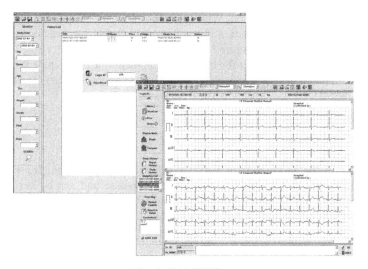

Fig. 3. EAMS Viewer

2.1 EAMS Modules

The EAMS was designed using Unified Modeling Language (UML) and is composed of main five modules, and the optional HIS Gateway, which is required only if the system is integrated with HIS. The architecture of the EAMS is represented in Figure 1 and the modules comprising it are as follows:

ECG Equipment: ECG instrumentation. Bionet's CardioCare 2000 and CardioTouch 3000, which support automatic ECG analysis, were tested with the system.

Acquisition Server: The acquisition server is connected with an electrocardiograph, an archiving server and the database. It retrieves the ECG work-list from the archiving server and acquires raw ECG data and ECG automatic analysis data from the ECG equipment. It matches the ECG data with the patient information obtained from the archiving server. Then it transfers the parsed information, such as weight, age, automatic analysis data, equipment information and ECG exam information from the acquisition server to the EAMS database, converts the ECG information into a DICOM waveform and sends it on to the archiving server. Figure 2.

Archiving Server: This server retrieves the ECG work-list from Radiology Information System (RIS) or from HIS, when EAMS is integrated with HIS, and sends it to the acquisition server upon request. After a patient's ECG examination, the archiving server retrieves the raw ECG data from the acquisition server, saves it and then communicates the path of the saved data to EAMS database. In addition, the archiving server monitors and controls the entire EAMS system. For example, the administrator can add or delete users' ID's by means of the archiving server.

Viewer: When the EAMS viewer is opened, it displays a list of un-read ECG examinations. User can search the EAMS database using keywords and can make an interpretation of the ECG examination. When the user selects an examination from the list, the viewer displays the examination's waveform signal and interpretation reports. The EAMS viewer is represented Figure 3.

All the EAMS modules except for the ECG equipment one, were implemented using C++ based on the Windows operating system, and are interconnected by means of the TCP/IP protocol.

2.2 EAMS Workflow

An example of the ECG examination workflow can be seen in Figure 4. All ECG information is archived centrally in the EAMS database and can be saved in local clients by physicians for further discussion and analysis. ECG data conforms to the DICOM waveform standard and can therefore be used for communication with other hospitals which have a standardized DICOM waveform system.

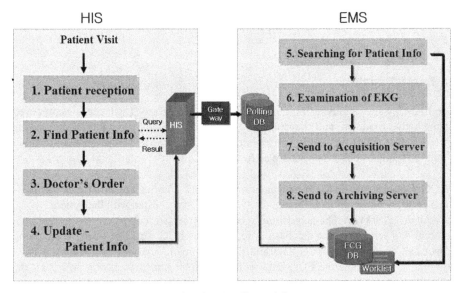

Fig. 4. EAMS Workflow

3 Data and Database Modeling

The ECG information model conforms to the DICOM waveform standard, which is represented in Figure 5, and the EAMS database schema (Figure 6) was designed taking into account this standard, as well as hospital medical care circumstances and the ECG characteristics for future ECG KDD systems.

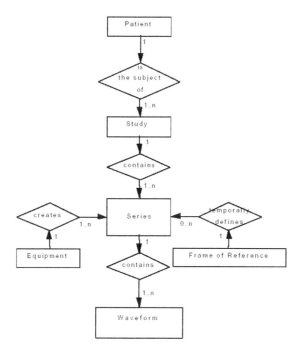

Fig. 5. DICOM Waveform Information Object Definition

Our initial conceptual model of the EAMS database had to be updated several times, due to ECG characteristics' considerations. The resulting model consists of 8 tables modeled to form a relational database linked by primary and secondary keys, and normalized to eliminate modification anomalies. The tables perform two functions. The five primary tables contain the following information:

Patient Table: patient information.
Study Table: supplementary examination data.
Waveform Table: specific ECG characteristics such as sampling frequency, channel information and ECG QRST information for future ECG KDD systems.
Results Table: information which has been confirmed by ECG specialists.
Results Modify Table: information concerning results which have been modified.

The other two supplementary tables, which store information that supports data entry for the purpose of system management contain the following information:

HIS Log Table: message file transferred from HIS.
User Table: information on the users who have been granted access to the EAMS database including their authorizations.

In addition, there exists a Normal Result Table which supports physicians' interpretation templates.

The EAMS database was created using Microsoft SQL Server 2000 and ODBC was used as a procedural language. Information in the EAMS database can be accessed via the search screen, and viewed using the EAMS viewer. Physicians and ECG specialists can write reports and confirm them.

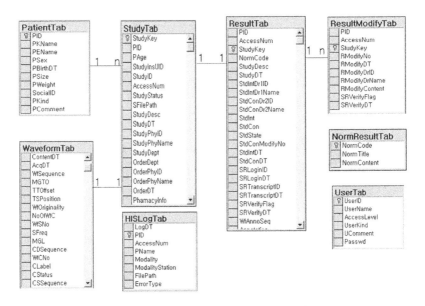

Fig. 6. EAMS Database Schema Design

4   Conclusion

In this study, we developed the EAMS partly based on the DICOM Waveform standard and modeled the EAMS database in order to take into account future ECG KDD systems. The EAMS, which we proposed, constitutes a useful tool for the acquisition and management of ECG waveforms. The EAMS also constitutes a useful counterpart for ECG KDD systems, because EAMS supports the DICOM waveform standards and because of the ECG characteristic EAMS database design.

Moreover, it is noteworthy that the EAMS can also provide a paperless solution for the handling of ECG information, which can liberate doctors from the complexity associated with the management of the current paper ECG charts.

5 Discussion

We developed the EAMS based on the DICOM waveform format, however we did not use the DICOM waveform protocol for interfacing with the ECG equipment, because existing ECG equipment does not conform to this protocol. Also, the use of Extensible Markup Language (XML) was not considered in this paper. Further effort is therefore needed in order for XML to be used for communicating ECG relational information to other hospitals, and for the interfacing of ECG KDD systems with EAMS.

References

1. W.J. Clancey, E.H. Shortliffe (eds.),.: Readings in Medical Artificial Intelligence - The First Decade: Addison-Wesley. (1984)
2. Krzysztof J. Cios(Eds.).: Medical Data Mining and Knowledge Discovery: Physica-Verlag, (2001)
3. Digital Image and Communications in Medicine: NEMA Standards Publication, 2001
4. H. K. Huang, D.Sc., FRCR (Hon.).: PACS: Picture Archiving and Communication Systems in Biomedical Imaging: VCH Publishers. (1996)
5. S Ombrato et al.: An Open System for Managing Long-Term ECG Recordings: Computers in Cardiology, IEEE, Vol. 27. (2000) 653-656
6. Taddei A., Carpeggiani C. et al.: Development of an electronic medical record for patient care in Cardiology: Computers in Cardiology, IEEE, Vol. 24. (1997) 641-644
7. I. Chouvarda, N. Maglaveras, C. Pappas, A. Boufidou: An Integrated Environment for ECG Processing: Medinfo, IOS Press, (1998) 986-989
8. Maglaveras N. et al.: IHIS: An Integrated Hospital Environment Linking via LAN ICU with PACS and Biochemical Laboratories: Computers in Cardiology, IEEE, (1996) 589-592
9. Mavromatis A. et al.: Integrated Cardiological Database Environment: Computers in Cardiology Proceedings, IEEE, (1994) 521-524

The Conceptual Basis of WITH, a Collaborative Writer System of Clinical Trials

Paola Fazi[1], Daniela Luzi[2], Fabrizio L. Ricci[3], Marco Vignetti[1]

[1]Dip. di Biotecnologie Cellulari e Ematologia, Unversità Roma – La Sapienza,
Via Benevento, 6, 00161 Rome, Italy
{Fazi,Vignetti}@bce.med.uniroma1.it
[2]ISPRI-CNR, Via dei Taurini, 19, 00185 Rome, Italy
luzi@isrds.rm.cnr.it
[3]Ist. Scienze Neurologiche (sez. Catania), V.le R. Margherita, 6,
95123 Catania, Italy
ricci@isrds.rm.cnr.it

Abstract. The paper illustrates the conceptual basis of the system WITH (Write on Internet clinical Trials in Haematology) which supports the collaborative writing of a clinical trial document. The requirements of this system have been defined analysing the writing process of a clinical trial and then modelling the content of its sections together with their logical and temporal relationships. This analysis generates a semantic network. The system WITH is based on XML mark-up language, and on a relational database management system. This choice guarantees: a) process standardisation; b) process management; c) efficient delivery of information-based tasks; and d) explicit focus on process design.

1 Introduction

The clinical guideline is used in daily medical practice when the related result of a clinical trial (CT) is successful. A CT is "any investigation in human subjects intended to discover or verify the clinical, pharmacological and/or pharmacodynamic effects of a product [...] with the object of ascertaining its safety and/or efficacy" [1]. The test of a CT is carried out only when an ad hoc committee has given its approval. This is based on the evaluation of a document (CT text), defined as "a written description of a trial of any therapeutic, prophylactic, or diagnostic agent conducted in human subjects, in which the clinical and statistical description, presentation and analyses are fully integrated into a single report" [1]. The writing of a CT document is a complex activity based on the collaboration of a team, which participates in the writing committee, generally working under the supervision of someone in charge of planning and co-ordinating the writing of the different sections of a CT. The physician responsible for the CT proposal has to control that the text is coherent and consistent in its parts also according to the rules of "good medical practice".

A. Colosimo et al. (Eds.): ISMDA 2002, LNCS 2526, pp. 86-97, 2002.

The GIMEMA (Italian Group for Haematological Disease of Adults) involves about 100 Italian centres and joins EORTC (European Organisation for Research and Treatment of Cancer). GIMEMA defines and manages several CTs active at the same time. It is therefore interested in developing a system which helps to define a new CT and write the related CT document based on standard procedures, and to re-use parts of ongoing or already closed CTs. We have developed the WITH (Write on Internet clinical Trials in Haematology) system which supports the editing of a CT. The aim of the WITH system is to help the end-user to write the CT text guiding him/hem in the preparation of standard and/or mandatory sections, controlling the internal consistency of the text and finally improving its diffusion on the network according to different views. This system is based on technologies integrating Relational DataBase Management System (RDBMS) with the XML mark-up language.

In this paper, however, our attention is focused on the conceptual basis useful to develop the WITH system. In section 2 we describe the work hypothesis on which our model is based together with the categorisation used in solving the problem of collaborative writing. In section 3 we describe the semantic network as the conceptual basis of the WITH system by means of tables containing the CT structure and the help information sources, as well as by means of state transaction, PERT diagrams and UML schema.

2   Preliminary Considerations

In the literature many studies have drawn attention on clinical guidelines (CGs). Various models have been used to represent CGs in their algorithmic parts, for example using flowchart [2], Arden syntax [3], state transition diagram [4], decision table [5], etc. It is however worth noting that CTs are different from clinical CGs. In order to obtain a correct evaluation of the CT investigation, a CT has to be rigidly followed; while CGs contain recommendation to improve the treatment. A structural description of the CT document has to respect the rules of "good clinical practice" and to determine the behavior of each participant in the test.

Currently XML is asserting itself as an exchange format, to represent and disseminate the knowledge contained in a CG (for instance [5,6,7,8]), and also because it facilitates the interoperability among different systems. We have adopted XML in the representation of the CT document.

The existing theories on collaborative writing are focused on the categorisation of the organisational patterns used by the collaborative writers. These categories are related to writing activities [9.10], writing strategies [9.11], rule subdivision [9], document control methods [9]. In our analysis we take these categories into consideration. Our experience has however showed that there is a dynamic and constant changing of roles and strategies carried out during the process of negotiation and communication typical of a collaborative writing. We have the advantage to know in advance the resulting text. Therefore, we have privileged the analysis of the correlation between the different sections of the CT and their segmentation according to criteria we are going to describe below. Organisational and collaborative strategies, which influence the draft of the text, are analysed through the direct observation of the clinical practice. For instance the physician who has elaborated the proposal outline of a new CT is generally responsible for it having determined, alone or in a team, the main parts of the document (objectives of the trial, statistical consideration, evaluation criteria and endpoints). This first phase is therefore very centralised and hierarchically controlled. Once these sections are defined, the drafting activities and their organisation are less rigid: people participating in this phase are more independent on both the content and the scheduling of the single sections.

3 The Model Adopted

The standardisation of CTs, considered as a minimum set of information mandatory for the description of the clinical and diagnostic investigation as well as for its approval, is a process, which has reached an advanced phase, but is not yet completed. The standardisation is limited by the differences existing among CT typologies, which present their own characteristics according to the type of investigation phase (I, II, III and IV steps) and to the type of study (randomised or not randomised). Besides these objective differences, there are other variations, which depend on the writing process of any type of text. Each CT text has its own feature, is subjected to customisations and variants related to a specific medical school, or is the result of the collaboration between different competencies (i.e. physician and statistician) or between different healthcare unites. Finally a CT is also subject to variations resulting from emerging needs, such as the ethical issue, which in recent years is becoming increasingly important.

Based on these considerations, which derive from the analysis of a meaningful number of CTs already developed by GIMEMA, we identify and suggest a standard structure of a CT document represented in the sections of table 1. The section names are related to the topics needed to describe a CT. It is possible to add new paragraph and subparagraphs, modify their order or change their titles, etc.

For the development of the WITH system we have taken into account the requirements necessary for:

a) editing the text based on a standard structure of a CT document, which is at the same time flexible enough to allow the user to change the structure, add new paragraphs, modify their order or change their titles, etc.;

b) guaranteeing the uniformity and the consistency of the document text;

c) facilitating the co-operation and the collaborative writing and monitoring the CT writing;

d) re-using the text (protocol libraries, data dictionary, etc.) and in particular re-using the sections which form the textual description of other CTs currently under test or already tested;

e) modeling the connection existing between the different sections, paragraphs and subparagraphs, in order to generate a hypertextual document;

f) managing the information related for instance to case record forms, to the healthcare structure suitable to perform CTs, etc.;

g) defining differentiated views of the CT, each one tailored on a specific type of user.

The requirements a) and b) imply an analysis of the sections and of their relations; the requirement c) implies the definition of a writing strategy; the requirements d), e), f), and g) imply the definition of the help information sources to write and to browse a CT document.

To fulfil these requirements we use a semantic network [12], which provides a formal description of a CT document together with the identification of their help information sources. The following nodes and edges compose this semantic network.

The nodes are:

- the sections (table 1);
- the elements composing a section (i.e.: laboratory tests, clinical criteria, etc.);
- the external systems (i.e.: standard texts, legacy systems, etc.).

The edges that represent different relationships between the nodes are as follows:

- The relationship "bound" represents a connection of logical-semantic coherence, which indicates that the different sections are closely interdependent. This means that between these sections there must be a consistency of both data and knowledge. This relationship admits the transitive and symmetric properties, which represent the close relationship among all the sections linked. For instance the sections "objectives of the trial" and "criteria of evaluation" have to be written by the same person or team because each objective is assessed through the measurement of well-defined evaluation parameters.
- The relationship "knows" represents a connection of both logical-semantic and temporal coherence. The sections connected by this relationship have to be written in a sequential way, according to the order of the edge direction. This means that different single writers may write these sections. Nevertheless the description of the randomisation procedure (contained in the section "patient registration") has to be written for instance consistently with and after the definition of the patient's eligibility (contained in the section "patient selection criteria").
- The relationship "equivalence" represents a loose connection of logical-semantic coherence, characterised by the presence of the same data, which has to be reported in different sections of the document. However there is a different information view of the same data reported in the document. For instance the list of the laboratory tests contained in the paragraph "required clinical evaluations, laboratory tests and follow up" corresponds to the list of fields of the communication form (paragraph: "Forms and procedures for collecting data"), which will report the result of the corresponding laboratory test.
- The relationship "belongs" represents the existence of an element composing a section. For instance the element of the section "Required clinical evaluations, laboratory tests and follow up" is equal to a component of the list of the laboratory tests.
- The relationship "uses" represents the existence of a standard text, the possibility of re-using a textual description, of accessing the information from other systems. For instance the paragraph "Ethical considerations" is based on a standard text.
- The relationship "implies" represents the connection between conceptual elements of different sections. For instance a particular clinical patient selection criteria is obtained by performing a well-defined laboratory test.

- The temporal relationships "after/before" and "together" represent the order to write the single sections of a CT document.

These relationships connect together the CT sections; the relationship "uses" connects a section with an external system; the relationship "belongs" connects a section with a single element; the relationship "implies" connects the elements of two or more sections.

The relationships "bound", "knows", "implies", "uses", and "belongs" are primitives. The relationships "belongs" and "equivalence" are isomorphic. The relationship "after/before" is equivalent to the relationship "knows"; the relationship "together" is equivalent to the relationship " bound ".

In this paper we are not going to describe the semantic network [12], but we illustrate the results of the semantic network analysis according to particular aspects: the section relation, the writing strategy and the help information sources for writing and browsing.

Table 1: The clinical trial structure

§	Section name
1	Background and introduction
2	Objectives of the trial
3	Patient selection criteria
4	Study / trial design
5	Therapeutic regimens, expected toxicity, dose modifications
6	Required clinical evaluations, laboratory tests and follow up
7	Criteria of evaluation
8	Endpoints
9	Patient registration
10	Forms and procedures for collecting data
11	Reporting adverse events
12	Data flow
13	Statistical considerations
14	Quality of life assessment
15	Cost evaluation
16	Data monitoring committee
17	Quality assurance
18	Ethical Considerations
19	Administrative responsibilities
20	Trial insurance
21	Publication policy
22	References

3.1 The Analysis of Sections and Their Relations

In the analysis of the sections and their relations we consider two problems: the manifold randomisation and the uniformity and consistency of a CT document.

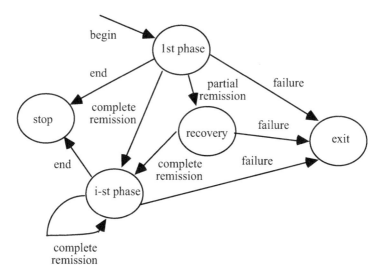

Fig. 1: The state transaction diagram

The study of a therapy may test different alternative paths, which may produce different randomisations. During a CT enactment, the patient may find him/herself in different states represented by the state transaction diagram of the fig. 1. The patient's healthcare process is composed by different phases. (In fig. 1 "i-st phase" represents the state related to the enactment of a generic phase.) Each phase implies the execution of a therapy cycle as well as a set of laboratory texts, used to monitoring the patient healthcare conditions. At the end of each cycle the patient can be in partial remission, or in complete remission, otherwise the therapy has failed. In case of partial remission, there is a recovery phase (state "recovery"), that is the therapy cycle aims to reach the patient's complete remission. There are two CT exit states: a) *stop*, when the patient has a positive response to the entire CT; and b) *exit*, when the therapy cycle has not been successful. Each phase implies a randomisation and therefore there is a repeated structure which is composed by manifold subparagraphs of the sections "Patient selection criteria" (section 3), "Patient registration" (section 9) and "Statistical considerations" (section 13). It is necessary to store data on different events (partial remission, complete remission, failure, etc.). The type of randomisation guides the composition of single sections. According to the number of randomisations, the system runs the state diagram for each possible combination of the patient's therapy response (partial remission, complete remission, failure) to each CT phase (1st phase, i-st phase and recovery) and suggests the structure of sections 3, 9, 13 in terms of subparagraphs.

The analysis of CTs has also led to the identification of 'key information' (the instance of an element node), which can be contained in specific sections. The uniformity and the consistency of the text are guaranteed by the use of key information within the different sections. These consistencies represent the relationships "knows", "equivalence" and "implies" of the semantic network. This key information is represented as a XML element to be inserted within the text, using well-defined attributes. The tagged key information represents a guide in the composition of a 'well formed' paragraph also under the perspective of the completeness and consistency of its content.

Considering the semantic network properties, we have:

- Let E_1, E_2 be two element classes, let S_1, S_2 be two section classes such that **belongs**(E_1,S_1) and **belongs**(E_2,S_2) and **implies**(E_1,E_2); then **equivalence**(S_1,S_2).

  If two sections are described by a different element and these elements are linked by the relationship "implies", there is an "equivalence" relationship between the two sections.

- Let e_1=**instance_of**(E_1) and e_2=**instance_of**(E_2) and **implies**(e_1,e_2), let s_1=**instance_of**(S_1) and s_2=**instance_of**(S_2) and **equivalence**(s_1,s_2), then **belongs**(e_1,s_1) implies **belongs**(e_2,s_2).

  If a CT section is described by a specific key information, the "equivalent" section is described by a well-defined key information.

These proprieties make it possible to write a CT text in a uniform and consistent way. If during the writing of the section s_1 we have inserted the key information e_1, in writing the section s_1 the system reminds the writer to insert the key information e_2.

The set of key information linked by the instances of "implies" relationship contributes to define a data dictionary and in particular this set represents the metadata needed to identify the CT in a univocal way. This set is stored in relational DB. The scheme of this DB is shown in fig. 2 by using the standard language UML, useful to describe the conceptual model of a DB [13].

The DB entity "statistical considerations" is the abstraction of the instances of "statistical considerations" element class of the semantic network. The same is also valid for "patient selection criteria", "clinical criteria" and "laboratory tests". The DB association "implies" between two DB entities (for example, E_1 and E_2) is the abstraction of the instances of the relationship implies (E_1,E_2). By means of the entities "kind of healthcare structure" and "performance procedure" and related associations ("executes" and "performances"), we store the specific information about the laboratory that carries out the test and how it is performed. This information is needed during the CT enactment.

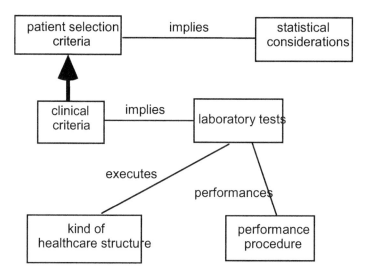

Fig. 2: The UML scheme

3.2 The Definition of the Writing Strategy

The time scheduling related to the writing of a CT is shown in fig. 3 by means of PERT diagram, obtained from the analysis of temporal relationships.
This analysis is based on the following semantic network properties:

- Let S_1, S_2 be two section classes, then **bound**(S_1,S_2) implies **together**(S_1,S_2). If there is a "bound" relationship between two sections, these sections must be written together.
- Let S_1, S_2 be two section classes, then **knows**(S_1,S_2) implies **after**(S_1,S_2).
  If there is a "knows" relationship between two sections, these sections must be written in cascade.
- Let S_1, S_2 be two section classes, then **equivalence**(S_1,S_2) implies **after**(S_1,S_2).
  If there is an "equivalence" relationship between two sections, these sections must be written in cascade.

Since the CT structure is standard, it can be modified even if it is defined only once: the user may add new paragraphs, modify their order, etc. In this case the PERT diagram is changed by the writing order of two or more sections. This is performed run-time as soon as the CT document structure is modified. By means of the PERT diagram it is possible to monitor the CT writing process and to advise the user to write a specific section.

The sections 2, 7, 8 and 13 describe the fundamental information of the CT and therefore have to be elaborated together as they are closely interdependent. They are the starting points for the drafting of section 3 and 4. The fundamental sections of the CT are now written, the other ones are generally drafted in an autonomous way. Each writing activity is performed by a group of people; it is necessary to manage the different versions of the CT, which represent the 'history of the document' and report the author's modified sections. Useful aids to collaborative writing are also the scheduling of a work plan (workflow) of the CT compilation, where the tasks of each editor can be reported together with the scheduled deadlines, as well as the management of e-mails exchanged by the different text authors.

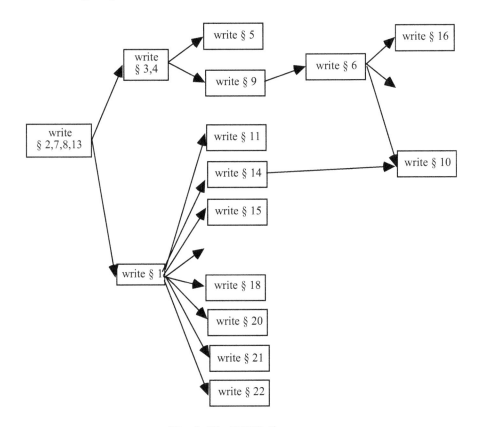

Fig. 3: The PERT diagram

3.3 The Definition of the Help Information Sources for Writing and Browsing

Writing a CT document is not an easy task and the style of writing is an intrinsic ingredient of the entire writing process. This process has some section writing activities that can be routine and pre-programmed. Others are more creative, however they have to follow specific rules and constraints, often contained in previous texts. These are the starting points that can be greatly modified. Therefore even if the system helps the writing in terms of re-use and advise, the experience and skills of a writer play an important role in a CT design.

The editing of a new CT is embedded within the medical activities conceptually related to the development of ongoing or already closed CTs, to guidelines used in a specific clinical praxis, to the results of laboratory and pharmaceutical research, which need a wider investigation. The complex process of writing a new CT can be facilitated by accessing libraries of CTs, and guidelines, data dictionary and databases of scientific papers, by the retrieval of information which can be stored and modified according to the specific requirements of the new CT. The analysis of the CTs has also drawn attention on parts of standard texts. The table 2 (related to the relationship "use") indicates the help information source for each section.

Table 2: The types of help information sources

$\S$	Help typology
2	DB of CTs
4	WF library
7	DB of criteria of evaluation classified for pathology
10	DB of forms DB of clinical data elements
11	DB of standard text
12	DB of standard text
14	DB of standard text
16	DB of addresses
17	Standard text
18	Standard text
19	DB of addresses
20	Standard text
21	Standard text
22	DB of references

The re-use of a section or of a part of it is based on the identification of a text stored in a DB or on the choice of a standard text. This means that the query definition is based on the key information belonging to the related section. Analysing the semantic network properties, we have:

- Let S_i a generic section class, let H_i a generic help class, let E_j a generic element class such that **belongs**(E_j,S_i) and **uses**(S_i,H_i).
- Let $s_i=$**instance_of**(S_i) and $h_i=$**instance_of**(H_i) and $e_j=$**instance_of**(E_j) such that **belongs**(e_j,s_i) and **uses**(s_i,h_i).

The system suggests a query based on a set of query clauses, whose generic element is a couple of the kind $< E_j, e_j>$ (element name and value). The user defines the logical operators for this clauses (and, or, etc.). This query is performed on the DB h_i. For each section s_i the semantic network and the CT key words (that is, the values of elements common to the main sections) make it possible to propose already prede-fined texts eventually to modify.

4 Conclusions

The WITH system integrates the technologies of RDBMS with the use of XML [14]. This choice is mainly connected with the need of an efficient management of CT libraries in terms of efficient storage, fast access, data integrity, security, etc. The WITH system guarantees: a) the process standardisation; b) the process management; and c) the efficient delivery of information-based tasks, the explicit focus on process design. Function libraries developed using MICROSOFT, ADO™ e XML-DOM™ components compose the system. The content of a generic CT is represented using a XML schema, composed by about 150 element types. The WITH system is available on the GIMEMA Intranet by Explorer™.

We are now working on the extension of WITH functionalities improving in particular the workflow editor to describe the "trial design" section. We have already developed at a prototype level a system which permits the description of a WF using a WF library, automates the procedures for the management of case record forms, patient registration and eligibility [14]. WITH is now in a β-test phase carried out by a selected group of GIMEMA, the first results are encouraging.

References

1 Guideline for good clinical practice. Available at http://www.eortc.be/documents.
2 Quaglini S, Stefanelli M, Lanzola G, Caporusso V, Panzarasa S.: Flexible guideline-based patient careflow systems. Artif. Intell. Med., 2001.
3 Hripcsak G, Ludemann P, Pyror TA, Wigertz OB, Clayton PD.: Rationale for the Arden Syntax. Comput. Biomed. Res., 1994.
4 Sugden B, Purves IN, Booth N, Sowerby M.: The PRODIGY Project - the Interactive Development of the Release One Model. Proceed. of AMIA Symp, 1999.
5 Shiffman RN, Karras BT, Agrawal A, Chen R, Marenco L, Nath S.: GEM: a proposal for a more comprehensive guideline document model using XML. J Am Med Inform Assoc, vol. 7, n. 5, 2000.
6 Dart T, Xu ., Chatellier G, Degoulet P.: Computerization of Guidelines: Towards a Guideline Markup Language. Proceed. of Medinfo, IOS Press, 2001.
7 Greenes RA, Boxwala A, Sloan WN, Ohno-Machado L, Deibel SR.: A framework and tools for authoring, editing, documenting, sharing, searching, navigating, and executing computer-based clinical guidelines. Proceed. of AMIA Symp, 1999.
8 Dubey AK, Chueh H.: Using the extensible markup language (XML) in automated clinical practice guidelines. Proceed. of AMIA Symp, 1998.
9 Flower LS, Schriver KA, Carey L, Haas C, Hayes J.R.: Planning in Writing: the cognition of a constructive process. Technical report, Centre for the Study of Writing, University of California, Berkeley, 1989.
10 Posner IR.: A study of collaborative Writing. M.SC. Thesis. Department of Computer Science, University of Toronto, 1991.

11 Ede L, Lunsford A.: Singular Texts/Plural Authors: Perspectives on Collaborative Writing. Carbondale, Illinois: Southern Illinois University Press, 1990
12 Fazi P, Luzi D, Ricci FL, Vignetti M.: A system definition to support collaborative writing of clinical trials. Proceeding of Information Society (IS 2001), 2001.
13 Foler M.: UML distilled. Addison-Wesley, 1997.
14 Fazi P, Luzi D, Manco M, Ricci FL, Toffoli G., Vignetti M.: WITH: a system to write clinical trials using XML and RDBMS. Proceeding of SCAMC 2002 (in print).

Problems of the Model Choice in Classes of Mendelian Inheritance Models

Bernd Jäger and Karl-Ernst Biebler

Institut für Biometrie und Medizinische Informatik, Ernst-Moritz-Arndt-Universität
Rathenaustraße 48, D - 17 487 Greifswald

Abstract. Model choice problems are looked at in classes of Mendelian inheritance models. Already for small allele numbers the model classes get very extensive. Statistical methods don't suffice for the decision for an inheritance model. It is necessary to look at parent-child relationships. Effects of a faulty model choice on the data evaluation are discussed.

1   Introduction

The population genetic models looked at in the following describe inheritance according to Mendel's theory and belong to the classic knowledge fund of genetics. Their application field has been extended to molecular genetics.

If a restriction lengths polymorphism is regarded as genetic marker, for example, then its distribution has to be described in the watched population.

In case that the genotypes are observable, the interpretation of the data not causes difficult problems. Allele frequencies are statistically estimated according to the gene counting method. This estimator is unbiased, effective in the sense of the statistical estimation theory and polynomial distributed. Confidence estimations of allele frequencies also being able to be calculated with that.

However, in more complex situations, it may not be possible to identify alleles uniquely from the banding patterns. Different genotypes may correspond to the same phenotype. It is required now to find a suitable inheritance model.

In this paper, aspects of the model choice are looked at from the combinatorial and statistical view.

In case one locus and three alleles all inheritance models are listed. Data concerning the ABO blood groups are used to find all statistically permitted 3-alleles models out. Then is argued that the observation of parent - child relationships is indispensable for the model choice.

Effects of a faulty model choice on the data evaluation are discussed.

2   Notations of Inheritance Models

Only one-locus models are looked at. $A_1, \ldots, A_k$ denote the alleles associated to the locus. The probabilities $p_1 = P(A_1), \ldots, p_k = P(A_k)$ deliver the genotype probabilities

A. Colosimo et al. (Eds.): ISMDA 2002, LNCS 2526, pp. 98-104, 2002.
© Springer-Verlag Berlin Heidelberg 2002

$$P(A_i A_j) = \begin{cases} p_i^2 & ;i = j \\ 2p_i p_j & ;i \neq j \end{cases}.$$

There are $n = k\,(k+1)/2$ different genotypes if $A_i A_j$ and $A_j A_i$ are identified. Every disjoint partition $\{T_1, ..., T_s\}$ of the set of genotypes defines an inheritance model. The $T_1, ..., T_s$ are called phenotypes. The probability of a phenotype is the sum of the probabilities of the underlying genotypes and therefore a function of the allele probabilities.

In case $k=2$, the alleles $A_1 = A$ and $A_2 = B$ with $p = P(A)$ and $1-p = P(B)$ may combined to genotypes AA, AB and BB. There are exact 5 disjoint partitions of the set of genotypes, listed in Table 1 together with the related phenotype probabilities.

Table 1. List of all Mendelian inheritance models with two alleles

No	phenotypes	phenotype probabilities	remarks
1	AA, AB, BB	p^2, $2p(1-p)$, $(1-p)^2$	all genotypes are observable
2	(AA,AB), BB	$p^2 + 2p(1-p)$, $(1-p)^2$	A is dominating B
3	AA, (AB, BB)	p^2, $2p(1-p) + (1-p)^2$	B is dominating A
4	(AA, BB), AB	$p^2 + (1-p)^2$, $2p(1-p)$	heterozygote is observable
5	(AA, AB, BB)	1	model degenerated

3   Size of Model Classes

Each number n of genotypes defines a set of inheritance models, which will be called class n. In the sense of model choice, the number k of alleles should be fixed first.

Table 2. All splits of n = 6 and of n = 7

No	n = 6	n = 7	remarks
1	6	6 + 1	
2	5 + 1	(5 + 1) + 1	splits of n = 7,
3	4 + 2	(4 + 2) + 1	derived from
4	3 + 3	(3 + 3) + 1	the splits of
5	4 + 1 + 1	(4 + 1 + 1) + 1	n = 6
6	3 + 2 + 1	(3 + 2 + 1) + 1	
7	2 + 2 + 2	(2 + 2 + 2) + 1	
8	3 + 1 + 1 + 1	(3 + 1 + 1 + 1) + 1	
9	2 + 2 + 1 + 1	(2 + 2 + 1 + 1) + 1	
10	2 + 1 + 1 + 1 + 1	(2 + 1 + 1 + 1 + 1) + 1	
11	1 + 1 + 1 + 1 + 1 + 1	(1 + 1 + 1 + 1 + 1 + 1) + 1	
12		7	trivial split
13		5 + 2	additional
14		4 + 3	splits
15		3 + 2 + 2	

What is about the size of class n, n = k (k + 1)/2 ? The answer is simple for k = 2. It is given in Table 1. One gets the size of class n as the number of different disjoint partitions of a set of n elements in two steps:

-   Determine all split of n into positive summands $n_1, ..., n_s, n_1 + ... + n_s = n$, where the n_i are natural numbers again.
-   Every split is identified with a disjoint partition of the set of n genotypes. The numbers of identical partitions are calculated by means of combinatorics.

Table 3. Disjoint partitions of the set of 6 genotypes without regard to the order: 203 Mendelian inheritance models

type	disjoint partitions of the set of genotypes with regard to the order	identical disjoint partitions	disjoint partitions of the set of genotypes without regard to the order
1	$\begin{pmatrix} 6 \\ 6 \quad 0 \end{pmatrix}$	all different	1
2	$\begin{pmatrix} 6 \\ 5 \quad 1 \end{pmatrix}$	all different	6
3	$\begin{pmatrix} 6 \\ 4 \quad 2 \end{pmatrix}$	all different	15
4	$\begin{pmatrix} 6 \\ 3 \quad 3 \end{pmatrix}$	2! (3 twice)	10
5	$\begin{pmatrix} 6 \\ 4\,1\,1 \end{pmatrix}$	2! (1 twice)	15
6	$\begin{pmatrix} 6 \\ 3\,2\,1 \end{pmatrix}$	all different	60
7	$\begin{pmatrix} 6 \\ 2\,2\,2 \end{pmatrix}$	3! (2 tree times)	15
8	$\begin{pmatrix} 6 \\ 3\,1\,1\,1 \end{pmatrix}$	3! (1 three times)	20
9	$\begin{pmatrix} 6 \\ 2\,2\,1\,1 \end{pmatrix}$	2! 2! (2 twice and 1 twice)	45
10	$\begin{pmatrix} 6 \\ 2\,1\,1\,1\,1 \end{pmatrix}$	4! (1 four times)	15
11	$\begin{pmatrix} 6 \\ 1\,1\,1\,1\,1\,1 \end{pmatrix}$	6! (1 six times)	1

With these details the size of class n is calculated. The determination of all splits of a natural number is a historical mathematical problem and up till now generally unsolved. Table 2 demonstrates a recursive method which can be programmed and delivers for the number of splits being interested here. In case n = 6 there are 11 types of splits.

From combinatorics is known, there are

$$\binom{n}{n_1 \ n_2 \ \ldots \ n_s} = \binom{n}{n_1}\binom{n-n_1}{n_2}\cdots\binom{n_s}{n_s}$$

choices of n_1 times phenotype T_1, n_2 times phenotype T_2, ..., n_s times phenotype T_s in n observations. The split $1 + 1 + 1 + 1 + 1 + 1$ of $n = 6$ (cp. Type 11 in Table 2) occurs 6! times. On the other hand, there are 6! permutations of 6 elements. Consequently, there is 6! / 6! = 1 disjoint partition of the set of six genotypes into six phenotypes (which are identical to the genotypes) without consideration of the order.

Table 3 demonstrates, the size of class n = 6 is 203. In other words: In the case of three alleles there are 203 Mendelian inheritance models.

For different genotype numbers, Table 4 indicates the size of the related classes of Mendelian inheritance models.

Table 4. Size of classes n of Mendelian inheritance models

number of genotypes n	disjoint partitions of the set of genotypes without regard to the order	remarks
2	2	
3	5	2-allele model
4	15	
5	52	
6	203	3-allele model
7	877	
8	4140	
9	21 147	
10	116 101	4-allele model

4   Statistical Aspects of Model Choice

The possibilities and the limits of statistical methods of the model choice shall be discussed at the example of the ABO blood group system. In the classical ABO-system, there are three alleles A, B and O and four phenotypes A = (AA, AO), B = (BB, BO), AB = (AB) and O = (OO). Two of the phenotypes are genotypes.

A sample of size N = 21 104 serves as data for the statistical model choice. The observed numbers are #A = 9123, #B = 2987, #AB = 1269 and #0 = 7725 [2].

Criterion is the chi-squared test of goodness of fit with significance level 0.05 in connection with a maximum-likelihood estimation of the unknown allele probabilities according to the inheritance model under test.

Four phenotypes are found. All 81 inheritance models corresponding to the partitions of 6 into at least four summends (Table 2, Table 3) are of interest.

The examination confines itself on the 45 models type 9 from Table 2. The phenotypes of these models correspond to the ABO-system. Since the data can be assigned to the phenotypes on 4! = 24 possibilities, 24 * 45 = 1080 parameter calculations and model tests become necessary. More than 40 models fit the data, 17 of them better as the ABO-system. The best fitting model is given in the Table 5.

As one sees, a model decision is not possible with statistical tools.

5   Parent – Child Relationship

Everyone of the data fitting models in the example is in contradiction to observed parent-child relationships. The ABO-system is the only exception and thus the only valid model. Consequently, discussions of parent-child relationships are essential in genetic model choice.

The argumentation shall be introduces briefly. The best fitting model to the data is given by the phenotypes (A_3A_3), (A_1A_2), (A_1A_3, A_2A_2) and (A_1A_1, A_2A_3), cp. Table 5. It is different from the ABO-system: There are two phenotypes which are genotypes at the same time. The homozygotes becomes identified, (A_3A_3) with (O,O). Let be A_1 the A-allele, A_2 the B-allele. The phenotype (A_1A_3, A_2A_2) then corresponds with genotypes (AO) and (BB) contrary to the ABO-system. Let be A_2 the A-allele, A_1 the B-allele. Then the argumentation is similar.

The best fitting model is false. Consider the mating of phenotypes "O" x "O". With regard to the underlying genotypes,

A_1A_1 x A_1A_1

A_1A_1 x A_2A_3

A_2A_3 x A_2A_3

are possible. Type "O"-parents can have A_1A_2 (that means "AB") children contrary to the reality.

Table 5. The best fitting model. The name of the phenotype was chosen according to the ABO-name of the related observations.

name	phenotype	observations	Chi-square
"B"	(A_3A_3)	2987	0.00113
"AB"	(A_1A_2)	1269	0.00003
"A"	(A_1A_3, A_2A_2)	9123	0.00168
"O"	(A_1A_1, A_2A_3)	7725	0.00068
Sum		21 104	0.00352

6   Conclusion

To identify a feature as a hereditary feature, the choice of an inheritance model is required. Because of the large number of the models to be checked this can be problematic.

At the data evaluation of genetic studies one distinguishes three situations.

- The inheritance model is not involved in the calculations. Mistakes in the model choice lead to misinterpretation of the results.

  To identify a observable property to be a marker for a certain disease, several risk measures are available. For a genetic result interpretation only it is important to know that the property looked at is hereditary.

- The calculation method is based on the inheritance model. Different models yield different calculation results for the same data.

  One compares the calculated allele frequencies from Table 6.

- The interpretation of the data is based on the inheritance model. A wrong model leads to observational bias.

  Take for example linkage analysis. Lod scores are calculated from the numbers of recombinant and non-recombinant haplotypes in the informative pedigrees. They do not depend from the inheritance model. The double heterocygotes are informative. But the identification of an individuum as heterocygote depends on the inheritance model. Table 6 demonstrates this for the ABO-system and the wrong but best fitting model. Figure 1 illustrates the part y of the heterocygotes in a population as function of two independent allele frequencies p and q.

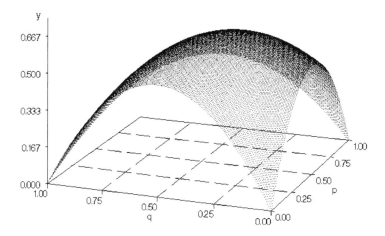

Figure 1. Part y of the heterocygotes in a population as function of two independent allele frequencies p and q.

Table 6. The subsets of heterocygotes (grey) in the population are different with respect to the AB0-system and the wrong but best fitting model

	phenotypes						allele frequencies
	"A"		"B"		"AB"	"0"	
classical model	AA	A0	BB	B0	AB	00	$p=P(A)=$ 0.2874
	p^2	$2pr$	q^2	$2qr$	$2pq$	r^2	$q=P(B)=$ 0.1064
	0.0825	0.3472	0.0113	0.1285	0.0611	0.3650	$r=P(0)=$ 0.0642
best fitting model	A_2A_2	A_1A_3	A_3A_3		A_1A_2	A_1A_1	A_2A_3	$x=P(A_1)=$ 0.5713
	y^2	$2xz$	z^2		$2xy$	x^2	$2yx$	$y=P(A_2)=$ 0.0526
	0.0027	0.4295	0.14		0.0600	0.3262	0.0395	$z=P(A_3)=$ 0.3761

References

1. Vogel, F., Motulsky A.G.: Human genetics. Springer-Verlag, Berlin Heidelberg New York (1976)
2. Helmboldt, W., Prokop, O.: Die Bestimmung der AB0-Genfrequenzen mittels der Maximum-likelihood-Methode und anderer Verfahren anhand forensischer Blutgruppenbestimmungen in Berlin. Blut 4 (1958) 190-201
3. Biebler, K.E.,Jäger, B.: Punkt- und Konfidenzschätzungen von Allelwahrscheinlichkeiten. In: Simianer, H. et al(eds.): Biometrische Aspekte der Genomanalyse. GinkgoPark Mediengesellschaft, Gützkow (1996)
4. Ott, J.: Analysis of Human Genetic Linkage. The Johns Hopkins University Press, Baltimore (1991)

Computational Modeling of the Cardiovascular System After Fontan Procedure

Eun Bo Shim[1], Chan Hyun Youn[2], Thomas Heldt[3], Roger D. Kamm[4], Roger G. Mark[3]

[1] Department of Mechanical Engineering, Kumoh National University of Technology,
Kumi, Kyungbuk 730-701, Republic of Korea
simeb@kumoh.ac.kr
[2] School of Engineering, Information and Communication University,
Taejeon, Republic of Korea
chyoun@icu.ac.kr
[3] Harvard-MIT Division of Heath Science and Technology,
Cambridge, MA 02139, USA
{thomas,rgmark}@mit.edu
[4] Biological Engineering Division, Massachusetts Institute of Technology,
Cambridge, MA 02139, USA
rdkamm@mit.edu

Abstract In this study, a computational method is presented to simulate the hemodynamics of patients after the Fontan procedure. The short-term feedback control models are implemented to assess the hemodynamic responses of the patients exposed to stresses such as gravity or hemorrhage. To construct the base line state of the Fontan model, we assume an increase in venous tone, an increase in heart rate, and an increase in systemic resistance all of which are based on clinical observations. For the verification of the present method we simulate a lower body negative pressure (LBNP) test and hemorrhage (20% blood volume loss). Both simulation results are compared to experimental data from the literature. Furthermore, it is shown that cardiac output decreases when the shunt resistance increases.

1. Introduction

The Fontan procedure was originally proposed for patients with tricuspid atresia [1]. Since then, it has been used in a variety of cardiac malfunctions, with a low risk of mortality and significant clinical improvement [2]. There are two types of Fontan procedures: cavopulmonary and atriopulmonary. The former has a flow path from the venae cavae directly to the pulmonary artery. In the latter type blood passes through the right atrium to the pulmonary artery with the right ventricle bypassed. In this study we concentrate on the atripulmonary type.

Many clinical experiments have been performed to investigate the hemodynamics of patients after the Fontan procedure, but there have been only a few published computational studies [3, 4]. Pennati et al. [3] have developed a computer model to represent the homodynamics in patients after the cavopulmonary procedure. They provided detailed numerical results on the systemic and the pulmonary circulation.

A. Colosimo et al. (Eds.): ISMDA 2002, LNCS 2526, pp. 105-114, 2002.

However, their model included no control system which is important when considering the dynamic response to stresses such as exercise, cold or heat stress, and hemorrhage. In these cases the short-term control plays an important role in the regulation of circulation.

In this study we implement a computational model to assess the hemodynamics of patients after a Fontan procedure. For the simulations, we used a lumped parameter model with six compartments closely resembling the previous work by our groups [5]. The mechanical properties of the cardiovascular system are modulated by two feedback control loops.

The results of the present model are compared with existing clinical data for verification of the method presented. We also calculate LBNP interventions and hemorrhage stress for Fontan patients and normal subjects. These results are compared with existing clinical data.

2. Hemodynamic Model Description

2.1 Hemodynamic Model for Normal Case

We utilize a lumped parameter model to simulate the cardiovascular system. The heart and circulation are represented in terms of electric circuit analogues. The entire model consists of six compartments: the left ventricle, the systemic arteries, the systemic veins, the right ventricle, the pulmonary arteries, and the pulmonary veins (Fig. 1). The pumping action of the heart is modeled by time varying ventricular compliances. Transmural pressure across the pulmonary capacitances varies according to intra-thoracic pressure, whereas the bias pressure P_{bias} at the systemic venous capacitance is used to simulate LBNP. Its value is set to zero except during the LBNP simulation.

The equations governing the hemodynamics of the cardiovascular system are derived from the pressure-flow relation to each node. Flow rate into and out of each node is determined by the pressure difference across the resistance between nodes. Application of Kirchhoff's law to the lumped parameter hemodynamic model leads to a resulting matrix equation as follows:

$$d\mathbf{p}/dt = \mathbf{Ap} + \mathbf{b} \qquad (1)$$

Here $\mathbf{p}$ is the vector of compartment pressures, $\mathbf{A}$ represent the time constants for exchange between compartments, and $\mathbf{b}$ is the input to the system. Starting with an estimated set of pressures, we can get the next set of pressures by solving the above set of the linear differential equation. We utilize a fourth-order Runge-Kutta scheme to solve the set of ordinary differential equation. Parameter values used in the present hemodynamic model are based on our previous paper [5] and are represented in Table 1. In this table, each compartment is characterized by an inflow resistance R_i with a unit of peripheral resistance units (PRU, mmHg·s/ml), a compliance C with a unit of ml/mmHg, a volume at zero transmural pressure V_0 (zero pressure filling volume, ZPFV) with a unit of ml, and an outflow resistance R_o.

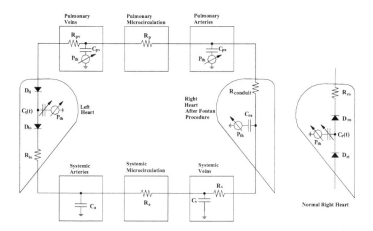

Fig. 1. Schematic of a lumped parameter model of the circulation after Fontan procedure.

Table 1. Summary of the hemodynamic parameters for normal case.

Compartment	R_i (PRU)	R_o (PRU)	C (ml/mmHg)	V_0 (ml)
Left heart	0.01	0.006	0.4 ~ 10	15
Systemic arteries	0.006	1.0	1.6	715
Systemic veins	1.00	0.025	100	2750
Right heart	0.025	0.003	1.2 - 20	15
Pulmonary arteries	0.003	0.08	4.3	90
Pulmonary veins	0.08	0.01	8.4	490

Total blood volume	V_{tot} = 5000 ml
Heart rate	72 beats/min
Thoracic pressure	-4 mmHg

2.2 Hemodynamic Model After Fontan Procedure

After a Fontan procedure, there is no right ventricular function. Since it has been documented that the right atrium plays an important role in the cardiovascular system of patients after atrio-pulmonary bypass [6], the right heart is modeled as a right atrial compartment (Fig. 1) after the Fontan procedure. The flow resistance due to bypass conduit is modeled by a resistive element between the atrium and the pulmonary arteries.

To construct the baseline state of Fontan model, we assume the following hemodynamic changes after Fontan procedure according in accordance with clinical observations:

Increased venous tone:
Kelly et al. [7] observed a 33% decreases in forearm venous capacitance in Fontan patients. On the basis of this data, we assume the same amount of decrease in overall venous capacitance after Fontan procedure.

Increased heart rate:
Heart rate in Fontan subjects increases compared with that of normal subjects by 3.2% - 33% (average 18%) [7]. We assume an 18% increase in heart rate after the Fontan procedure.

Increased systemic resistance:
A 20% increase in systemic resistance after Fontan procedure has been documented [8] and implemented in our model.

3. Control Model Description

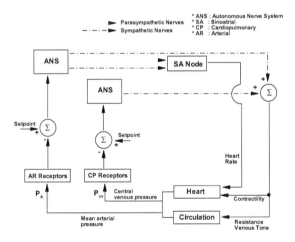

Fig. 2. Diagram of the control system in the present model

We implement the short-term regulation of cardiovascular system that consists of the two major neural mediated cardiovascular reflexes: the arterial baroreflex and the cardiopulmonary reflex. These reflex loops mediate the short-term control mechanisms of arterial pressure and blood volume respectively, acting over seconds to minutes. As shown in Fig. 2, the baroreflex receptors in the carotid sinus and the cardiopulmonary receptors in the right atrium transmit pressure variations to the ANS (Autonomic Nervous System). A fast parasympathetic reflex arc acting through the vagus nerve tightly controls heart rate while slower sympathetic fibers modulate the strength of ventricular contraction and peripheral vascular tone in addition to a slower modulation of heart rate. The effects of the reflexes on control variables such as heart rate, heart contractility, peripheral resistance, and venous tone are described using the beat-to-beat model proposed by DeBoer et al. [9].

4. Results and Discussion

4.1 Computational Results of Patients After Fontan Procedure

Kelly et al. [7] have published the hemodynamic differences between normal subjects and Fontan subjects. They found that the increased venous tone (decreased venous capacitance) for Fontan patients might be the cause of the impaired cardiac output.

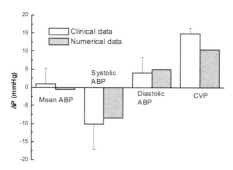

Fig. 3. Comparison of hemodynamic changes between the normal and the subject after the Fontan procedure. In here $\Delta(\bullet) = (\bullet)_{Fontan} - (\bullet)_{normal}$ and HR, ABP, CVP represent heart rate, arterial blood pressure, and central venous pressure, respectively.

Flow resistance due to the bypass conduit (or pressure drop through the conduit) depends on the fluid dynamical state through the shunt and the flow pathway of the Fontan operation. According to Shachar et al. [8], the pressure drop through the conduit in the Fontan operation is about $0.3 - 4.3$ mmHg (average 2.3 mmHg). We assume that the pressure drop due to the conduit resistance is about 2.3 mmHg. Clinical and numerical results of some hemodynamic variables are depicted in Fig. 3.

4.2 LBNP Simulation for Normal Subject and Patients After the Fontan Procedure

The results of the LBNP simulations for both normals and Fontan subjects are shown in Fig. 4 along with experimental data taken from [7].

LBNP results for Fontan patient group are shown in Fig. 5. Less decrease in CVP during LBNP is observed in Fontan patient group. As explained in Kelley et al. [7], this is due to the increase of venous tone after Fontan procedure. In the numerical results we can also find the same phenomenon (see Fig. 4(d) and Fig. 5(d)).

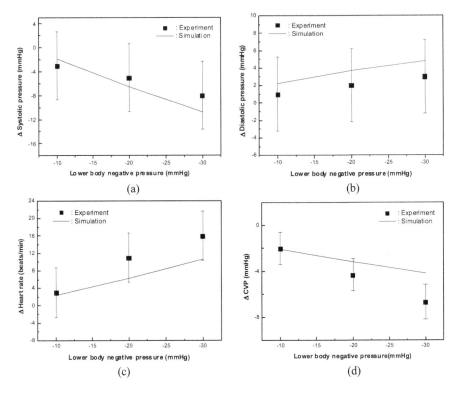

Fig. 4. Hemodynamic changes during graded LBNP for the normal model. In here $\Delta(\ \bullet\ )$ = $(\ \bullet\ )_{LBNP} - (\ \bullet\ )_{no\ LBNP}$. Changes in (a) systolic ABP, (b) diastolic ABP, (c) heart rate, (d) CVP.

4.3 Exposure to Hemorrhage

We simulate hemorrhage by a decrease in total blood volume in the model. Computed results for normal subjects are shown in Fig. 6 in case of 20% hemorrhage. The decrease in total blood volume causes the arterial blood pressure and the central venous pressure to decrease, which activates the baroreceptor reflex and the cardiopulmonary reflex system.

The systemic resistance modulated by the two reflex systems increases to reduce the increased blood pressure and volume. The present numerical results are compared with the experimental ones of vagotomized dogs in Fig. 6. Though there are some deviations in systemic resistance, the other hemodynamic values obtained from the present study agree well with the experimental ones [10] and the existing numerical data [11].

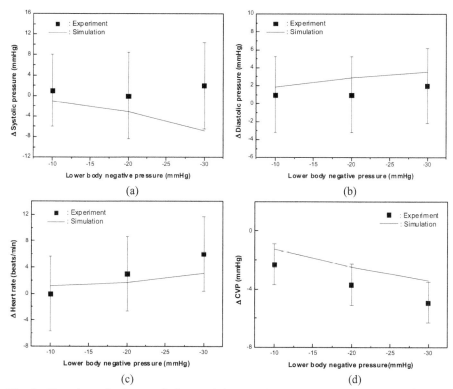

Fig. 5. Hemodynamic changes during graded LBNP for the Fontan model. In here $\Delta(\bullet) = (\bullet)_{LBNP} - (\bullet)_{no\ LBNP}$. Changes in (a) systolic ABP, (b) diastolic ABP, (c) heart rate, (d) CVP.

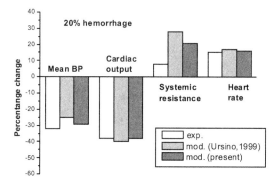

Fig. 6. Percentage changes in the hemodynamic variables after 20% hemorrhage case for the normal model.

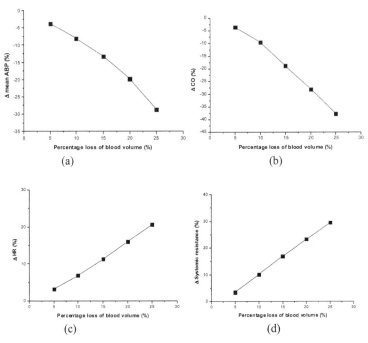

Fig. 7. Changes in hemodynamic parameters of a patient after the Fontan procedure as a function of blood volume loss. (a) Mean ABP (b) Cardiac output (c) Heart rate (d) Systemic resistance.

Results from the parametric study showing the effect of an increase in blood volume loss from 5% to 25% is shown in Fig. 7. Mean ABP and cardiac output decrease abruptly whereas heart rate and systemic resistance linearly increase as the blood volume loss increases.

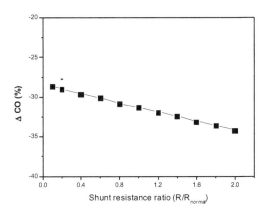

Fig. 8. Cardiac output changes of a patient after the Fontan procedure according to the shunt resistance.

4.4 Effect of the Conduit Resistance

Conduit resistance varies according to the fluid dynamical situation within the shunt. Fig. 8 shows a linear decrease in cardiac output when shunt resistance is increased. Doubling the resistance results in a 3% decrease of cardiac output.

5. Conclusions

In this study, we presented a computational model to simulate the hemodynamic states of patients after a Fontan procedure. The hemodynamic model for the Fontan patient group is constructed using a lumped parameter approach. To set the baseline state of the Fontan model, we assumed increased venous tone, heart rate, systemic resistance, and flow resistance due to the conduit. The proposed method includes the two control mechanisms, the arterial baroreflex and the cardiopulmonary reflex model. LBNP has been simulated and the results show good agreement with experiments. The increased venous tone in the Fontan model causes a smaller decrease of CVP during LBNP compared with the normal (non-Fontan) case. 20% hemorrhage results compare favorably with existing numerical results. We also conducted a parametric study in which blood volume is reduced successively. Mean ABP and cardiac output decrease abruptly whereas heart rate and systemic resistance increase linearly as blood volume is reduced. Numerical results of the effects of shunt resistance on cardiac output show a linear decrease in cardiac output as shunt resistance is increased.

References

1. Fontan, F., and Baudet, E., 1971, "Sugical repair of tricuspid atresia," *Thorax*, Vol. 26, pp. 240-248.
2. Gale, A. W., Danielsson, G. K., McGoon, D. C., and Mair, D. D., 1979, "Modified Fontan operation for univentricular heart and complicated congenital lesions," *J. Thorac. Cardiovas. Surg.*, Vol. 78, pp. 831-838.
3. Pennati G, Migliavacca F, Dubini G, Pietrabissa R, Fumero R, de Leval MR., "Use of mathematical model to predict hemodynamics in cavopulmonary anastomosis with persistent forward flow," *J Surg Res.* 2000 Mar;89(1):43-52.
4. Rydberg, A., Teien, D. E., and Krus, P., 1997, "Computer simulation in patient with total cavo-pulmonary connection: inter-relationship of cardiac and vascular pressure," flow, resistence and capacitance, *Med. Biol. Eng. Comput.*, Vol. 35, pp. 722-728.
5. Heldt T, Shim EB, Kamm RD, Mark RG., "Computational modeling of cardiovascular response to orthostatic stress," *J Appl Physiol* 2002 Mar;92(3):1239-54
6. Bull, C., de Leval M. R., and Stark, J., 1983, "Use of a subpulmonary ventricular chamber in the Fontan circulation," *J. Thorac. Cardiovas. Surg.*, Vol. 85, pp. 21.
7. Kelley, J. R., Mack, G. W., and Fahey, J. T., 1995, "Diminished venous vascular capacitance in patients with univentricular hearts after the Fontan operations," *American Journal of Cardiology*, Vol. 76, pp. 158-163.
8. Shachar, G. B., et al., 1982, "Rest and exercise hemodynamics after the Fontan procedure," *Circulation*, Vol. 65, pp. 1043-1048.

9. DeBoer, R. W., 1987, "Hemodynamic fluctuations and baroreflex sensitivity in humans: A beat-to-beat model," *American Journal of Physiology*, Vol. 253(22), pp. H680-H689.

10. Kumada, M., Schmidt, K., Sagawa, K., and Tan, K. S., 1970, " Carotid sinus reflex in response to hemorrhage," *Amer. J. Physiol.*, 243, H499-H504.

11. Ursino, M. and Innocenti, M, 1997, "Modeling arterial hypotension during hemodialysis," *Artificial Organs,* Vol. 21, 873-890.

Short- and Long-Term Statistical Properties of Heartbeat Time-Series in Healthy and Pathological Subjects

Paolo Allegrini[1], Rita Balocchi[2], Santi Chillemi[3], Paolo Grigolini[3,4,5], Luigi Palatella[4], and Giacomo Raffaelli[6]

[1] Istituto di Linguistica Computazionale del Consiglio Nazionale delle Ricerche, Area della Ricerca di Pisa-S. Cataldo, Via Moruzzi 1, 56124, Pisa, Italy. (paolo.allegrini@ilc.cnr.it)
[2] Istituto di Fisiologia Clinica del Consiglio Nazionale delle Ricerche, Area della Ricerca di Pisa-S. Cataldo, Via Moruzzi 1, 56124, Pisa, Italy.
[3] Istituto di Biofisica del Consiglio Nazionale delle Ricerche, Area della Ricerca di Pisa-S. Cataldo, Via Moruzzi 1, 56124, Pisa, Italy
[4] Dipartimento di Fisica dell'Università di Pisa and INFM, via Buonarroti 2, 56127 Pisa, Italy.
[5] Center for Nonlinear Science, University of North Texas, P.O. Box 311427, Denton, Texas, 76203-1427 USA.
[6] International School for Advanced Studies and INFM Unit, via Beirut 2-4, 34014 Trieste, Italy.

Abstract. We analize heartbeat time-series corresponding to several groups of individuals (healthy, heart transplanted, with congestive heart failure (CHF), after myocardial infarction (MI), hypertensive), looking for short- and long-time statistical behaviors. In particular we study the persistency patterns of interbeat times and interbeat-time variations. Long-range correlations are revealed using an information-based technique which makes a wise use of the available statistics. The presence of strong long-range time correlations seems to be a general feature for all subjects, with the exception of some CHF individuals. We also show that short time-properties detected in healthy subjects, and seen also in hypertensive and MI patients, and completely absent in the trasplanted, are characterized by a general behavior when we apply a proper coarse-graining procedure for time series analysis.

1   Introduction

In the last few years, time series analysis techniques have been applied to heartbeat sequences to detect long-range memory [1,2,3]. With these methods one can in principle distinguish between different statistical properties that may correspond to different pathophysiological condition. Another important goal of this analysis is to unravel the hidden control mechanisms responsible for the heartbeat dynamics. Indeed heart rate variability is influenced by the "competition" between sympathetic and parasympathetic nervous system activity as well as by

A. Colosimo et al. (Eds.): ISMDA 2002, LNCS 2526, pp. 115–126, 2002.

non-autonomic factors. Consequently, an analysis regarding different time scales can in principle disentangle the different contributions to the heart rate variability. In this work we use a recently developed technique for measuring long-range correlations called *Diffusion Entropy* (DE) [4,5,6]. We also focus on short-range time behavior and, using a coarse-graining procedure, we identify an objective resolution time for the measure of the interbeat distance. We use this results to compute the relative importance of the short-time dynamics with respect to the long-term one.

2   Materials and Methods

2.1   The Diffusion Entropy Technique

In order to process the data, the first step consists of a coarse-graining procedure on the RR time series. This strategy, shared also by other groups (see, for instance, Ref. [2]) makes a statistical treatment of the data possible.

We define a coarse-graining parameter s and we obtain a new series, namely

$$T_i(s) \equiv [T_i/s], \tag{1}$$

where T_i is the time distance between the ith and the $i - 1^{th}$ beat, $T_i(s)$ is the coarse-grained time series and $[\cdot]$ denotes the integer part. Equation (1) means that we preliminary divide the interbeat distance scale in several "boxes" of size s and we assign to all the interbeat distances lying in the same "box" the same value in the sequence $T_i(s)$. Next, we convert this series into a dichotomous sequence, setting $\xi_i = 1$ when $T_i(s) \neq T_{i-1}(s)$, and $\xi_i = 0$ if $T_i(s) = T_{i-1}(s)$. Finally, we generate several trajectories (labelled with the index l) for the variable x_l at "time" t, namely,

$$x_l(t) = \sum_{i=l}^{l+t} \xi_i. \tag{2}$$

Note that, for simplicity, we have omitted indicating the dependence on s. As shown in Ref. [4], if the sequence ξ_i is ergodic, then the probability distribution of the variable x as a function of t is expected to fit the scaling property

$$p(x,t) = \frac{1}{t^\delta} F\left(\frac{x}{t^\delta}\right), \tag{3}$$

with the "degree of anomaly" being measured by the distance of the scaling parameter δ from the standard value 0.5 corresponding to Brownian motion.

It is straightforward to prove that the Shannon entropy

$$S(t) = -\int_{-\infty}^{\infty} p(x,t) \ln(p(x,t)) \mathrm{d}x \tag{4}$$

of a process fitting the scaling condition of Eq. (3) yields

$$S(t) = A + \delta \ln(t), \tag{5}$$

where A is a constant, whose explicit form is not relevant for the ensuing discussion. This result is immediately obtained by plugging Eq. (3) into Eq. (4). The above method of evaluating the scaling parameter δ is called Diffusion Entropy (DE), and, as it will become clear later, this technique is more efficient than the calculation of the second moment of the probability distribution. Note that when the distribution density under study departs from the ordinary Gaussian case and the function $F(y)$ has slow tails with an inverse power law nature [4] the second moment is a divergent quantity. This diverging quantity is made finite by the unavoidable statistical limitation. In this case, the second moment analysis would be determined by the statistical inaccuracy, thereby leading to misleading conclusions, while the method based on Eq. (5) yields correct results [4,5].

2.2   Short-Time Analysis

Let us define the sequence $\{\tau_j\}$ as the distance between 1's in the series $\{\xi_i\}$. The authors of Ref. [4] studied the case where the probability distribution for τ decays as an inverse-power law with exponent $\mu > 2$. If τ_j were uncorrelated, then a simple expression would exists, linking μ and δ, namely

$$\delta = \frac{1}{\mu - 1} \ (\delta = 0.5 \text{ if } \mu > 3). \tag{6}$$

In our analysis we observe a strong discrepancy between the values of $\delta \approx 0.8$ and of $\mu \approx 5$, thus suggesting that the sequence of τ_j has a long time memory [6]. This is why we perform the normalized auto-correlation function of the sequence τ_j defined as

$$\Phi_\tau(j) = \frac{\langle(\tau_k - \langle\tau\rangle)(\tau_{k+j} - \langle\tau\rangle)\rangle}{\langle\tau_k^2\rangle - \langle\tau\rangle^2} \tag{7}$$

where $\langle\cdot\rangle$ is the arithmetic average, e.g.

$$\langle\tau\rangle \equiv \frac{1}{N}\sum_{k=0}^{N}\tau_k, \tag{8}$$

and N is the number of terms in the sum.

At this point we realize that for most data the correlation function $\Phi_\tau(j)$ actually decays as an inverse power law after an abrupt fall occurring at the transition from $j = 0$ to $j = 1$. The value at $j = 1$, defined as ϵ^2, exhibits a peculiar behavior as a function of the coarse-graining parameter s. We will show that this behavior is typical of all the groups, with the exception of transplanted patients and some CHF individuals.

2.3   RR Time Series

The RR series analyzed are taken from the *NOnLinear TIme Series AnaLysIS* (NOLTISALIS) archive. This data set is the result of the collaboration of several interdisciplinary Italian research centers. The data correspond to 50 patients classified in 5 groups of 10 subjects each: normal, hypertensive, post-MI, with congestive heart failure, and heart transplanted.

For each subject there are 24-hour Holter recordings, whose sample frequencies range from 128 to 1024 Hz, according to the type of pathology.

3   Results

3.1   Long-Term Analysis

The analysis performed with the Diffusion Entropy technique yields very accurate fits as shown in Figs. 1 and 2. The average results for each group of patients is shown in table 1.

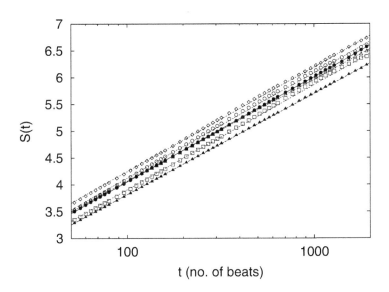

Fig. 1. Diffusion Entropy S(t) for healthy patients. The straights lines in log-linear scale represent best fits for Eq. (5)

As shown in table 1, the values of δ indicate very strong correlations for all the different groups. The CHF individuals, however, as previously shown in Ref. [2,6], are characterized by a somewhat smaller value. One of the main results of this paper is that, remarkably, the results from table 1 are independent of the coarse-graining parameter s. As we shall show later, this property can be accounted for by a simple intermittent model.

On the other hand, the coarse-graining parameter s becomes very important in evaluating the correlation function $\Phi_\tau(j)$. In fact, different values of s yield different series for τ, while a large/small coarse graining leads to higher/lower

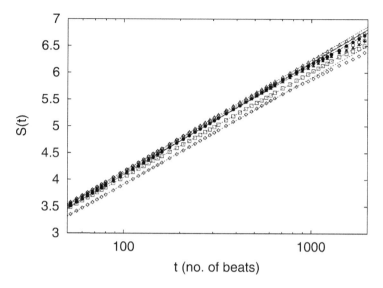

Fig. 2. Diffusion Entropy S(t) for patients hypertensive. The straights lines represent best fits for Eq. (5)

value for $\langle \tau \rangle$. We investigate the different correlation functions stemming from different coarse-graining values s. As earlier stated, in most cases the correlation function presents an abrupt drop going from $j = 0$ to $j = 1$. After this fast drop, it decays to zero very slowly, like an inverse-power law. In fact, the data are not clean enough to establish the inverse power law index with a good accuracy. This means that the DE is a much more efficient method to detect memory and much less ambiguous than the correlation function, and we can actually describe the meaning of δ making use of a general class of dynamical models. The correlation function $\Phi_\tau(j)$, on the other hand, depends on the details of the model and does not afford an easy way to derive it.

Table 1. Average value of δ for each group of patients

Group	$\langle \delta \rangle$
healthy	0.83 ± 0.02
CHF	0.80 ± 0.05
post-MI	0.85 ± 0.04
transplanted	0.86 ± 0.08
hypertensive	0.87 ± 0.02

The numerical form of the correlation function $\Phi_\tau(j)$ is

$$\Phi_\tau(j) = (1 - \epsilon^2)\delta_{j,0} + \epsilon^2 C(j). \tag{9}$$

Here $\delta_{j,0}$ denotes the Kronecker δ step, while the function $C(j)$ is a smooth function with the property $C(0) = 1$. We account for the long-term properties, namely second term in the r. h. s of (9), as follows. We hypothesize that the heartbeat rate, on a rather long time scale, undergoes trends of acceleration and deceleration of slopes α, whose duration length τ are asymptotically distributed with an inverse power law, with index μ'. We suppose that the consecutive trends are not correlated and consequenlty the scaling parameter δ is connected to μ' via [4]

$$\delta = \frac{1}{\mu' - 1}. \tag{10}$$

Here we sketch a proof of Eq. (10). First of all we define the distribution probability for the slope α, $f(\alpha)$. We make the simplifying and plausible hypothesis that this distribution has no infinite moments. This restriction does not apply to the τ-distribution, which has, on the contrary slow tails and diverging moments. Without loss of generality we assume the following form

$$\psi(\tau) = \frac{A^{\mu'-1}}{(A + \tau)^{\mu'}}, \tag{11}$$

where $A = \langle\tau\rangle/(\mu' - 2)$. During one single trend of acceleration or deceleration the position of the walker $x_l(t)$ is displaced by a quantity

$$z = \frac{|\alpha|}{s}\tau, \tag{12}$$

which is the number of times the walker crosses the "box boundaries" defined by the coarse-graining procedure on T_i. Consequently, we can write the probability of a displacement z that reads

$$p(z) = \int_0^\infty d\tau \int_{-\infty}^\infty d\alpha\delta\left(z - \frac{\alpha\tau}{s}\right)\psi(\tau)f(\alpha). \tag{13}$$

After many trends it is straightforward to see, e. g. along the lines of Ref. [8], that the movement of our walker is essentially equivalent to a process where a walker, at regular time distances of duration $\langle\tau\rangle$, walks by a quantity $\Delta x \sim z$, distributed as

$$\Pi(\Delta x) = \frac{s}{|\alpha|\langle\tau\rangle}\psi\left(\frac{s\Delta x}{|\alpha|}\right). \tag{14}$$

Since the function ψ has a long tail, this latter process, according to the Generalized Central Limit Theorem [9], results in a Lévy Flight, which is a stable process with diverging central moments. The difficulty of dealing directly with the distribution (14) is due to the fact that α is itself a stochastic variable.

However we can detect the asymptotic scaling property of the walker $x_l(t)$ by studying the first diverging moment of the distribution $p(z)$. To find this value we evaluate

$$\langle z^\gamma \rangle = \int_0^\infty p(z)z^\gamma dz. \tag{15}$$

The smallest value of γ for which this integral diverges, called $\hat{\gamma}$, defines the scaling δ via $\delta = 1/\hat{\gamma}$ [9]. Plugging Eq. (13) into (15), we obtain

$$\langle z^\gamma \rangle = \int_0^\infty dz \int_0^\infty d\tau \int_{-\infty}^\infty d\alpha\ \delta\left(z - \frac{\alpha\tau}{s}\right) \psi(\tau)f(\alpha)z^\gamma. \tag{16}$$

Integrating over z, this result can be written as

$$\langle z^\gamma \rangle = \left(\int_0^\infty \psi(\tau)\tau^\gamma d\tau\right) \cdot F_s, \tag{17}$$

where

$$F_s = \int_{-\infty}^\infty d\alpha \left(\frac{|\alpha|}{s}\right)^\gamma f(\alpha). \tag{18}$$

This means that only the first factor might make $\langle \tau^\gamma \rangle$ divergent, thereby implying that $\hat{\gamma} = \mu' - 1$ and proving Eq. (10). This also proves that δ *does not depend either on the coarse-graining parameter s or on the distribution of α*, which in fact contribute only to F_s.

We now establish an interesting connection with the two-walkers model of Ref. [6] as follows. We assume that the trajectory T_i is a zig-zag path. Each straight line of this path is determined by the slope α_j, which connects the persistency time τ_j to the coarse-grain parameter s, by

$$\alpha_j = \frac{s}{\tau_j}. \tag{19}$$

If the straight line portion of the zig-zag curve has length l_j, we have about $l_j\alpha_j/s$ identical values of τ_j. These are the pseudoevents of the two-walkers model of Ref. [6].

3.2   Short-Term Analysis

Of course this crude model can only describe the long-time regulation of the heartbeat dynamics and has to be supplemented with middle- and short-time corrections so as to take into account the abrupt fall corresponding to the first term in the r.h.s. of Eq. (9). Indeed short-term control mechanisms are due to the activity of the autonomic nervous system which presents a very short time scale.

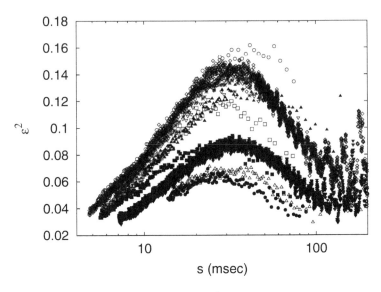

Fig. 3. Short-time correlation parameter ϵ^2 as a function of the coarse-graining resolution s for all the the healthy subjects. Two of them are plotted with a much higher number of points, to show both the subtle erratic dependence and the "continuous" one.

We use a short-time (local) perturbation model which does not destroy long-time properties, in a way that is similar to the point-like mutations affecting the long-range correlations in DNA sequences [10]. The value of ϵ^2 does in fact depend on the value of s and therefore we compute $\epsilon^2(s)$ in order to investigate the properties of these control mechanisms. Surprisingly enough, the function $\epsilon^2(s)$ show a quite universal feature for all healthy and hypertensive individuals: we observe a steep increase as s goes from few msec up to $s_{max} \cong 30$ msec where we have a maximum. After that we have a slow decrease until 200 msec. The most striking result is that, even if the maximum value is quite different among the various individuals, the values of s_{max} seems to be universal, the variability among different patients being lower than 5 msec. This result is shown in Fig.3. This feature is somewhat visible (always for $s_{max} = 30$ msec) also in post-MI or hypertensive patients (see Fig. 4) and even in some CHF ones, while it is completely absent in some CHF patients and in all the heart transplanted. Results for these latter groups are shown in Fig. 5.

To the best of our knowledge, the interpretation of s_{max} is not easily explained in physiological terms. With the due caution, we may intepret this scale as an intrinsic resolution for the assessment of the heartbeat rate from the control system. In other words there should be a natural coarse graining in the physiological determination of the interbeat time distance. The fact that this behavior is missing in the case of heart transplanted patients seems to imply the action of the autonomic system. Anyway, the measured timescales rule out

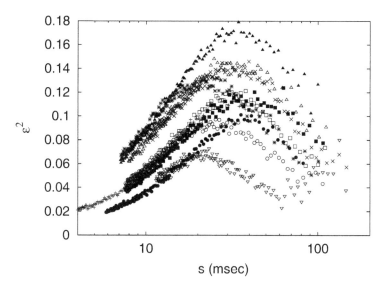

Fig. 4. Short-time correlation parameter ϵ^2 as a function of the coarse-graining resolution s for 5 hypertensive patients and 5 post-MI patients. We plot only half of these groups for plot clarity.

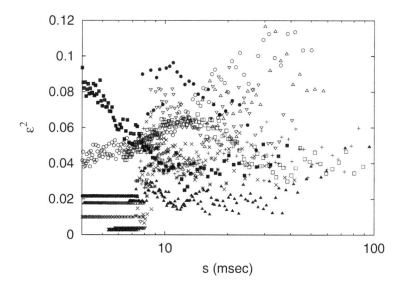

Fig. 5. Short-time correlation parameter ϵ^2 as a function of the coarse-graining resolution s for all 10 transplanted patients. The structure of the previous figures is absent.

the possibility that this maximum is due to the sampling rate of the measuring apparatus. We conclude that more work has to be done to explain this effect throughfully. Finally, from a methodological point of view we use this property to evaluate in an objective way a value for the parameter ϵ^2, which is a measure of the *regularity* of the interbeat time accelerations α during the trends of variation.

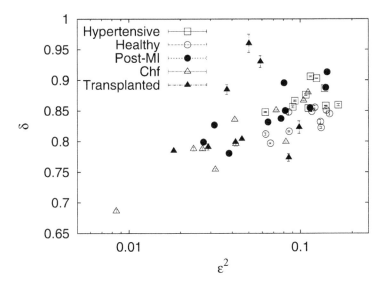

Fig. 6. Bidimensional plot of $\delta(\epsilon^2)$ for all the 50 subjects.

At this point, as done in Ref. [6], we can plot the value of δ, independent of our coarse graining, as a function of our objectively defined value of ϵ^2. The result is shown in Fig. 6. We recall that both parameters reflect *memory*, the former being associated with long-range fractal properties, and the latter with short-time persistency in the heart acceleration patterns. This latter behavior is certainly connected with multifractal properties, as reported e.g. in Ref. [11]. Arguably, the proposed treatment here proposed is more intuitive.

Fig. 6 shows the $\{\epsilon^2, \delta\}$ scatter plot for all 50 subjects. Even though there is no satisfactory statistical discrimination among groups, maybe due to a variety of factors like the limited number of patients, differences in illness seriousness and differences in therapy, we observe that healthy individuals are concentrated in a small portion of the graph, in agreement with the results of Ref. [6]. Hypertensive patients, too, have their peculiar region, characterized by an higher value of δ. Other pathologies seem to occupy broader regions. A significant portion of pathological individuals occupy the "healthy zone", and these may be associated to less serious conditions. Actually, preliminary results (unpublished) on an enlarged group of CHF patients seem to suggest a correlation between serious condition and the absence/distorsion of the $\epsilon^2(s)$ peak at 30 msec. These patients are also characterized by a smaller value of $\epsilon^2(s)$ and they are therefore mostly outside the "healthy" zone.

4 Conclusions

In conclusion, this study allows us to propose, on the basis of a simple statistical analysis, a series of conjectures to be accurately tested by further studies. The physiological long-range memory, probably due to a cascade of mechanisms at different timescales, can be characterized by two parameters, the scaling δ of the underlying infinite-memory process, and the weight ϵ^2, which gives information of the relative importance of this latter process versus short-time mechanisms. The presence of the 30 milliseconds peak of Fig. 3, which allows an objective definition of ϵ^2 seems to be physiological and corresponds to the presence of a fast control mechanism, which has to react in a time shorter than few heartbeats to properly explain the abrupt fall of the correlation functions. This control mechanism seems to act with a special time resolution: a "grid" of about 30 milliseconds. The absence, distorsion, or shift of this internal resolution may reflect a pathological condition and is often associated with a lower degree of long-time memory.

Finally, we stress that the coarse-graining procedure adopted herein yields results that are independent of the coarse-graining parameter, making this analysis robust. We believe that this analysis can be applied with success to a variety of time series with both long- and short-time structures, and even to nonstationary signals. Results stemming form our procedure may thereby provide additional information useful in many diagnostic and prognostic problems. In general, we envisage our procedure as an automatic classifier for those complex sequences that are not easily dealt with, using usual statistical learning methods. Applications may range from natural-language semantic classifiers based on *discourse dynamics* to predictors of catastrophic events [5].

Aknowledgements. We gratefully acknowledge financial support from the Army Research Office through Grant DAAD 19-02-0037. One of the authors (P. A.) acknowledges European Commission POESIA project (IAP2117/27572) for financial support. L. P. acknowledges ENEL Research Grant 3000021047 for support.

References

1. Shlesinger, M.F.: Fractal time and 1/f noise in complex system. Ann. NY Acad. Sci. **504** (1987) 214–228; Bassingthwaighte, J.B., Liebovitch, L.S., West, B.J.: Fractal Physiology. Oxford University Press, New York (1994)
2. Ashkenazy, Y., Ivanov, P.Ch., Havlin, S., Peng, C.-K., Goldberger, A.L., Stanley, H.E.: Magnitude and Sign Correlation in Heartbeat Fluctuations. Phys. Rev. Lett. **86** (2001) 1900–1903

3. Balocchi, R., Barbi, M., Carpeggiani, C., Chillemi, S., Di Garbo, A., Michelassi, C.: Complexity and Predictability of the Heartbeat Time Series in Transplanted Subjects. Int. J. Bifurcation and Chaos **7** (1997) 759–767

4. Grigolini, P., Palatella, L., Raffaelli, G.: Asymmetric Anomalous Diffusion: an Efficient Way to Detect Memory in Time Series. Fractals **9** (2001) 439–449

5. Allegrini, P. ,Grigolini, P., Hamilton, P., Palatella, L., Raffaelli, G., Virgilio, M.: Facing nonstationarity condition with a new indicator of Entropy Increase: the Cassandra Algorithm. In: Novak, M.N. (ed.): Emergent Nature. World Scientific, Singapore (2002) 173–184

6. Allegrini, P., Grigolini, P., Hamilton, P., Palatella L., Raffaelli, G.: Memory Beyond Memory in Heart Beating, a Sign of a Healthy Physiological Condition. Phys. Rev. E **65** (2002) 041926–041930

7. Signorini, M.G., Sassi, R., Cerutti, S.: Working on the Noltisalis Database: measurement of nonlinear properties in heart rate variability signals. In: Proc. of the 23th Annual Conf. of the IEEE-EMBS, Istanbul, Turkey, Oct 24-28 (2001)

8. Annunziato M., Grigolini, P.: Stochastic versus Dynamic Approach to Lévy Statistics in the Presence of an External Perturbation. Phys. Lett. A **269** (2000) 31–39

9. B. V. Gnedenko, B.V., Kolmogorov, A.N.: Limit Distributions for Sums of Independent Random Variables. Addison Wesley, Cambridge MS (1954)

10. Allegrini, P., Buiatti, M., Grigolini, P., West, B.J.: Fractional Brownian Motion as a Nonstationary Process: an Alternative Paradigm for DNA sequences. Phys. Rev. E **57** (1998) 4558–4567

11. Ivanov, P.Ch., Nunes Amaral, L.A., Goldberger, A.L., Havlin, S. Rosenblum, M.G., Struzik, Z.R., Stanley, H.E.: Multifractality in Human Heartbeat Dynamics. Nature **399** (1999) 461–463

An Index of Organization of the Right Atrium During Atrial Fibrillation: Effects of Internal Cardioversion

Vincenzo Barbaro[1], Pietro Bartolini[1], Giovanni Calcagnini[1], Federica Censi[1], Antonio Michelucci[2], and Samantha Poli[1,3]

1 Biomedical Engineering Laboratory, Istituto Superiore di Sanità,
Viale Regina Elena 299, 00161 Roma, Italy
{Barbaro, Bartolin, Giovanni.Calcagnini, Censi}@iss.it
2 Department of Internal Medicine and Cardiology, Univ. of Florence, Italy
michelucci@unifi.it
3 Department of Information and System Science, University of Rome, Italy
poli@dis.uniroma1.it

Abstract. Aim of this study is to investigate the effects of unsuccessful internal cardioversions on the propagation of the depolarization wavefronts in the right atrium during atrial fibrillation, by using an index of organization of endoatrial signals (electrograms). The organization was estimated by computing the percentage of points laying on the signal baseline (i.e., number of occurrences, NO). Electrograms were recorded by using a multipolar basket catheter. NO values were computed on two-second long windows, one just before and five just after unsuccessful shocks. We found that immediately after the shock there was an increase in the organization, which fades within few seconds after the shock delivery. Our data show that the proposed index provides the quantitative assessment of organization in the entire right atrium, and gives experimental support to the hypothesis that unsuccessful shocks cause a widespread extinction of electrical wavefronts, which regenerates after the shock.

1. Introduction

Atrial fibrillation (AF) is the most common, sustained arrhythmia that occurs in humans and presents a number of therapeutic choices, both pharmacologic and nonpharmacologic. A widely used nonpharmacologic therapeutic approach in patients with AF is the Low Energy Internal Cardioversion (LEIC), obtained either by external direct-current cardioversion or by catheter defibrillation. It is believed that successful AF termination by electric shock is related to the termination of reentrant propagating wave fronts [1]. It has been hypothesized that after unsuccessful shocks a reduction of propagation wavefront is achieved, followed by a regeneration of propagating wavefronts within few seconds. If that is so, a transient increase in the organization of bipolar electrograms should be observed.

The morphology of bipolar endocardial recordings during AF has often been studied in terms of 'organization'. Wells et al. [2] first gave criteria for scoring the organization of single bipolar recordings, and identified four types of AF. The organization is in turn related to the number of depolarization fronts entering the

A. Colosimo et al. (Eds.): ISMDA 2002, LNCS 2526, pp. 127-133, 2002.

recording site. The number of occurrences (NO), defined as the percentage number of points along the baseline of a single bipolar electrogram, turned out to reliably classify AF organization according to Wells' criteria [3].

Aim of this study is to investigate the effects of internal cardioversion energies on the wavelet propagation of the right atrium, by using an index of organization of endoatrial signals (electrograms). The study is based on the estimation of organization of electrograms obtained by a multipolar basket catheter (MBC) inserted in the right atrium.

2. Methodology

2.1 Experimental Protocol

Bipolar electrograms were obtained from MBC (Constellation, Boston Scientific, MA, USA) in the right atrium in 13 haemodynamically stable patients with documented persistent AF, selected a priori for LEIC. The MBC is composed of 64 platinum-iridium equally-spaced electrodes mounted on 8 flexible, self-expanding splines, 8 electrodes each spline (figure 1). Each spline is identified by a letter (from A to H), the electrodes on each spline are identified by numbers (from 1 to 8).

MBC was advanced via the left or right femoral vein. From the 64 electrodes, 32 bipolar electrograms were derived by combining electrodes 1and 2, 3 and 4, 5 and 6, 7 and 8, for each spline and were labeled A12, A34, ..., H78 (figure 1). These electrograms were filtered (pass-band 10-300Hz), digitized (1-kHz, 16 bit) and stored on magneto-optical disk, using a Bard Labsystem polygraph. Surface leads (I, II, III, aVR, aVL, aVF and V1) were also recorded.

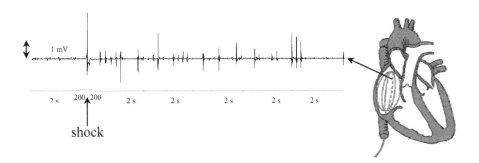

Figure 1. Sketch of the basket catheter inserted in the right atrium. One electrogram is shown, together with two-second long windows selected for the computation of NO. 200 ms immediately before and after each shock were excluded from the analysis

After a 10-minutes long basal monitoring, a step-up protocol was used for LEIC. It started with a nominal shock energy of 0.5 J, then increased at the following levels: 1, 2, 3, 5, 7, 10, 15 and 20 J. The procedure was stopped when a stable sinus rhythm was recovered (>1 minute). Two 6F decapolar catheters were used for the internal cardioversion: one with the distal tip positioned in the right atrial appendage; the other inserted into the coronary sinus.

2.2 Definition of Anatomic Locations

In order to find a relation between the electrophysiological properties associated to each bipole and the anatomical site of that bipole and to statistically compare the data from different patients, a definition of the anatomic locations was made. Fluoroscopically identifiable markers on the MBC (1 on spline A and 2 on spline B) furnished the orientation of the basket in the right atrium, while V-waves artifacts identified those bipoles close to the tricuspid valve circumference [4][5]. V waves artifacts were quantified in terms of ventricular signal-to-noise ratio (SNR_V). Signals with SNR_V lower than 10 dB were considered likely to come from bipoles close to the tricuspid valve region.

Right atrium was then divided into 32 anatomical regions obtained as follows: first, each spline has been associated to 8 anatomic 'vertical' regions of the atrium (figure 1) namely, anterior free wall (AFW), lateral free wall (LFW), postero-lateral free wall (PLFW), posterior free wall (PFW), posterior atrial septum (PAS), atrial septum (AS), tricuspid valve (TV) and anterior tricuspid valve (ATV). Second, each region was further divided into high (bipoles 1-2), mid-high (bipoles 3-4), mid-low (bipoles 5-6) and low (bipoles 7-8) segments (figure 2).

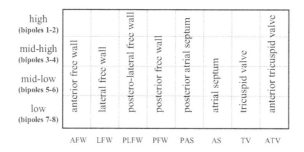

Figure 2. Definition of the 32 anatomic regions.

2.3 The Index of Organization of Endoatrial Recordings

We estimated the level of organization by computing the number of occurrences, NO as the percentage of points laying on the signal baseline. This parameter reliably classifies AF organization according to Wells' criteria based on the morphology of single bipolar atrial electrograms [2][3]. Wells' classification divides AF in 4 types: Type I (AF1), characterized by discrete, beat-to-beat, atrial electrogram complexes of variable morphology and cycle-length, separated by an isoelectric baseline free of perturbation; Type II (AF2), similar to Type I, but characterized by a not isoelectric baseline and by various perturbations; Type III (AF3), characterized by no longer detectable isoelectric segments are associated with discrete intervals and. Type IV (AF4) characterized by Type III atrial electrograms and by alternating electrogram periods consistent with Type I and/or II. Examples of AF1, AF2 and AF3 are shown in Figure 3.

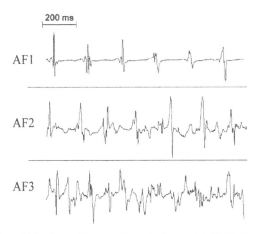

Figure 3. Examples of bipolar atrial recordings during atrial fibrillation: atrial fibrillation of Type I (AF1), Type II (AF2) and Type III (AF3).

After performing a signal amplitude normalization, the amplitude range was divided in 33 intervals (bins), and those points falling within the central bin were considered to belong in the baseline. The number of baseline points (i.e. points in the central bin) was divided by the total number of points in the segment, to obtain the percentage of baseline points (NO). Examples of APDF for AF1, AF2 and AF3 are shown in Fig. 4.

NO values were computed on 2 s long windows immediately before (NO_{before}) and after (NO_{after}) each shock. In order to avoid the shock artifact be included in NO computation, 200 ms immediately before and after each shock were excluded from the analysis (see figure 1). After the last unsuccessful shock, five sequential windows were selected in order to track the time course of the NO values (figure 1).

3. Results

All the patients were successfully cardioverted. Cardioversion energies ranged 3J-20J. The dynamic behavior of NO values, in one patient, 2 seconds before and five 2-second long windows after the last unsuccessful shock is shown in Figure 5. The 4

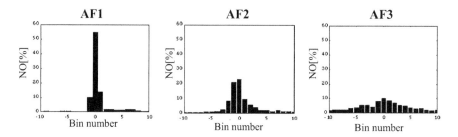

Figure 4. NO in the three types of AF. NO in AF1 is dominated by a large peak in the central bin; the NO for AF2 presents significant (populated) bins around the baseline; in AF3 the bins are spread out over a wide range around the baseline.

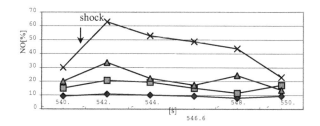

Figure 5. NO values evolution in one patient 2 seconds before and five 2-second long windows after the last unsuccessful shock. The 4 tracks correspond to NO values from the 4 bipoles of one spline of the MBC.

tracks belong to a spline located in the AFW. Note that a higher level of organization is reached immediately after the shock, while a decrease is then observed. Similar results have been obtained for the other patients.

Since the basal NO differs among the patients, in order to compare the effect of the last unsuccessful shock on NO in the 13 patients, we performed the following categorization: first, in each patient, we computed the differences between NO_{before} and NO_{after}, for each bipole. This difference was called ΔNO. Then the differences were categorized as:

-1   for $\Delta NO < -10$
0   for $-10 \leq \Delta NO \leq 10$
1   for $\Delta NO > 10$

These scores were then summed over the population, for each anatomical region. In this way we obtained a single score for each region, ranging from -13 to $+13$. For a given atrial region, a score of -13 would mean that all patients got a decrease in the organization greater than 10%, in that region, while an increase of organization in most of the patients would give values toward $+13$. These results are shown in figure 6. Positive scores prevail in most of the regions. In addition, the high and mid-high regions had increase in organization greater than the low and mid-low ones. In order to validate this methodology, we also computed the difference between two NO pre-shock values (NO_{before}), randomly chosen within the basal recording, and we

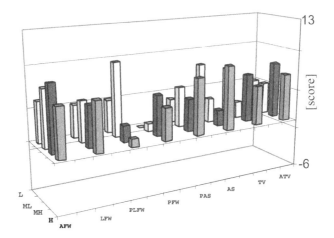

Figure 6. Scores summed over the population, for each anatomical region. Scores may have values from –13 to +13. See text for details.

categorized them according to the same criterion used for post-shock evaluation. Figure 7 shows these scores summed over the population, for each anatomical region. Note that the ΔNO scores are randomly distributed around zero. In addition, the high and mid-high regions had increase in organization greater than the low and mid-low ones

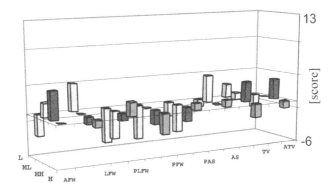

Figure 7. ΔNO scores computed between two successive NO_{before} summed over the population, for each anatomical region.

4. Discussion and Conclusion

The present study examined the time course of the effects of internal cardioversion energies on the wave fronts propagation in the right atrium immediately after the energy delivery by using an index of organization of atrial electrograms.

We found that the effect of the shock is an increase in the level of organization within 2 seconds immediately after the last unsuccessful shock in all right atrial regions. This effect appears to be transient, with restoration of original NO within 10 seconds. This finding suggests the idea that the electrical shock causes a widespread extinction of electrical wavefronts, which regenerate after the shock [1] and that the shock does not affect the organic substrate [6]. This result is consistent with our previous finding: when computed over 10 second long window, no significant differences are present in the average NO after the shock [7].

Since we found an increase of organization all over the right atrial region, it might be hypothesized that sub-threshold shocks delivered at specific sites (showing the most disorganized electrical activity) could provoke the wave fronts interruption over the critical mass of the myocardium. This will lead to a decrease in the patient discomfort and pain, which has limited the diffusion of automated atrial defibrillators, so far.

References

1. Prakash A, Saksena S, Krol RB, Philip G. Right and left atrial activation during external direct-current cardioversion shocks delivered for termination of atrial fibrillation in humans. Am J Cardiol 2001 May 1;87(9):1080-8
2. Wells JL, Karp RB, Kouchoukos NT, Maclean WAH, James TN, Waldo AL. Characterization of atrial fibrillation in man: studies following open-heart surgery. Pacing Clin Electrophysiol. 1978;1:426-438.
3. Barbaro V, Bartolini P, Calcagnini G, Censi F, Morelli S, Michelucci A. Mapping the organization of atrial fibrillation with basket catheters - part I: validation of a real-time algorithm. Pacing Clin Electrophysiol. 2001 Jul;24(7):1082-8.
4. Pitschner HF, Berkovic A, Grumbrecht S, Neuzner J. Multielectrode basket catheter mapping for human atrial fibrillation. J. Card. Elecrophysiol 1998; 9(8):S48-56.
5. Triedman JK, Jenkins KJ, Colan SD, et al. Multipolar endocardial mapping of the right heart using a basket catheter: acute and chronic animal studies. Pacing Clin Electrophysiol. 1997;20(1 Pt 1):51-9.
6. Everett TH, Li H, Mangrum JM, Mastrangelo C, Haines DE. The effects of atrial electrical remodeling on atrial defibrillation thresholds. Pacing Clin Electrophysiol 2001 Aug;24(8 Pt 1):1208-15
7. V Barbaro, P Bartolini, G Calcagnini, F Censi, R Macioce, A Michelucci. Effects of Internal Cardioversion on Electrophysiological Properties of the Right Atrium. Computers in Cardiology Conference 2001 Vol 28:301:304

Morphological Analysis of ECG Holter Recordings by Support Vector Machines

S. Jankowski[1], J. Tijink[2], G. Vumbaca[2], M. Balsi[2], G. Karpinski[3]

[1]Institute of Electronic Systems, Warsaw University of Technology,
ul. Nowowiejska 15/19, 00-665 Warsaw, POLAND
sjank@ise.pw.edu.pl
[2]Department of Electronic Engineering, University of Rome "La Sapienza"
via Eudossiana 18, 18-00184 Rome, ITALY
balsi@uniroma1.it
[3]Chair and Department of Internal Medicine and Cardiology, Central Teaching Hospital
ul. Banacha 1a, 02-097 Warsaw, POLAND

Abstract. A new method of automatic shape recognition of heartbeats from ECG Holter recordings is presented. The mathematical basis of this method is the theory of support vector machine, a new paradigm of learning machine. The method consists of the following steps: signal preprocessing by digital filters, segmentation of the Holter recording into a series of heartbeats by wavelet technique, support vector approximation of each heartbeat with the use of Gaussian kernels, support vector classification of heartbeats. The learning sets for classification are prepared by physician. Hence, we offer a learning machine as a computer-aided tool for medical diagnosis. This tool is flexible and may be tailored to the interest of physicians by setting up the learning samples. The results shown in the paper prove that our method can classify pathologies observed not only in the QRS alterations but also in P (or F), S and T waves of electrocardiograms. The advantages of our method are numerical efficiency and very high score of successful classification.

1 Introduction

The goal of this work is to present a new, complete toolbox for Holter ECG processing that can recognise the predefined shapes of heartbeats.

1. Given a complete filtered ECG Holter recording as input, the segmentation tool can divide it in a series of single heartbeats.
2. The support vector machine provides an adequate approximation of the waveform as a sum of Gaussian functions. The Lagrange multipliers in this approximation can substitute the discrete samples representing the signal.
3. A carefully chosen subset of these SVM parameters represents the heartbeat, or its part.

This processing stresses the characteristics of one single beat. The shape of one heartbeat contains a large amount of information about the conduction of the stimulus within the heart.

A. Colosimo et al. (Eds.): ISMDA 2002, LNCS 2526, pp. 134-143, 2002.

Our paper presents the preliminary results of applied technique and we show rather the promising effects than the validation of our algorithms studied on the large database. We worked on a database of ECG Holter records from the Department of Internal Medicine and Cardiology at the Central Teaching Hospital in Warsaw. The signals are digitised with 128 Hz sampling rate and filtered with a 514 coefficients digital FIR filter. The records are processed using filter banks to provide a segmentation of the signal into single heartbeats. Then each heartbeat is approximated by a continuous function representing the signal. From this approximation, meaningful parameters are taken to represent the single heartbeat. These parameters can be used as input for a classifier that can distinguish the beats in classes according to their shapes.

2 Mathematical Basis of Support Vector Machines

Support vector machine is an idea of optimal learning machine first formulated by Vapnik[1,2], support vector machine performs new ideas of supervised learning from examples. Let $X \subseteq R^n$ - the input space, Y - the output domain, e.g. for binary classification $Y = [-1, 1]$, for function approximation $Y \subseteq R$. A training set consists of a collection of training examples:

$$S = ((\mathbf{x_1}, y_1), (\mathbf{x_2}, y_2),...,(\mathbf{x_l}, y_l)) \subseteq (X \times Y)^l$$

l - number of examples, $\mathbf{x}$ - examples, y - their labels.

Given a linearly separable set S the optimal separating hyperplane $(\mathbf{w},b)$ solves the following optimisation problem:

$$\min_{\mathbf{w},b} (\mathbf{w} \cdot \mathbf{w}) \tag{1}$$

subject to

$$y_i((\mathbf{w} \cdot \mathbf{x}_i) + b) \geq 1, \quad i = 1,...,l \tag{2}$$

It realises the maximal margin hyperplane with the geometric margin $\gamma = 1/\|\mathbf{w}\|_2$. This problem can be solved by introducing Lagrange multipliers $\alpha_i \geq 0$ and a primal Lagrangian L:

$$L(\mathbf{w},b,\mathbf{\alpha}) = \frac{1}{2}(\mathbf{w} \cdot \mathbf{w}) - \sum_{i=1}^{l} \alpha_i[(y_i(\mathbf{w} \cdot \mathbf{x}_i) + b) - 1], \quad \alpha_i \geq 0 \tag{3}$$

The Lagrangian L has to be minimized with respect to the primal variables $\mathbf{w}$ and b and maximized with respect to the dual variables α_i. The dual form is the following:

$$L(\mathbf{w},b,\mathbf{\alpha}) = \sum_{i=1}^{l} \alpha_i - \frac{1}{2} \sum_{i,j=1}^{l} y_i y_j \alpha_i \alpha_j (\mathbf{x_i} \cdot \mathbf{x_j}) \tag{4}$$

Hence, the hyperplane can be described as a linear combination of the training points:

$$\mathbf{w}^* = \sum_{i=1}^{l} y_i \alpha_i^* \mathbf{x}_i \tag{5}$$

This expansion consists of only a small subset of data from the training set that correspond to non-zero Lagrange multipliers - these points are called the support vectors.

The regression problem can be seen as a classification into an infinite number of classes. In order to approximate functions, an ε-insensitive loss function will be used: The learning phase of the machine corresponds to fitting an elastic tube onto the training points. The training points are the data of the problem. It is possible that the chosen tube is so hard to adapt that some points will fail to fit in it and will lie outside. The slack variables ξ_i, ξ_i^*, have been introduced to deal with this case. The value of C determines how much deviations larger than ε are tolerated with respect to the flatness of the tube.

The key idea is to construct a Lagrange function from both the objective function and the constraints, by introducing a set of dual variables:

$$L = \frac{1}{2}\|\mathbf{w}\|^2 + C\sum_{i=1}^{m}(\xi_i + \xi_i^*) - \sum_{i=1}^{m}\alpha_i(\varepsilon + \xi_i - y_i + \langle \mathbf{w}, \mathbf{x_i}\rangle + b) - \sum_{i=1}^{m}\alpha_i^*(\varepsilon + \xi_i^* + y_i - \langle \mathbf{w}, \mathbf{x_i}\rangle - b) \quad (6)$$

$$- \sum_{i=1}^{m}(\eta_i\xi_i + \eta_i^*\xi_i^*)$$

The dual variables are $\alpha_i, \alpha_i^*, \eta_i, \eta_i^*$, and have to satisfy positive constraints $(\alpha_i, \alpha_i^*, \eta_i, \eta_i^* \geq 0)$. The primal variables are $\mathbf{w}, b$ and ξ_i, ξ_i^* . These last are the slack variables and η_i, η_i^* have been introduced to induce their positivity

We use the algorithm that quickly solves the support vector machine problem - sequential minimal optimisation (SMO) - extreme decomposition of the problem that involves two Lagrange multipliers only at any one step [4].

3 Segmentation

A Holter ECG recording is a continuous or discrete time signal composed of subsequent heartbeats. The QRS complex acts as a flag, an indicator of the presence of a heartbeat. Detection of the QRS complex (specifically, detection of the R peak of the QRS complex) in an ECG signal is a difficult problem since it can be subject to important modifications due to heart pathologies.

The wavelet transform provides an adaptive approach. As a wavelet is a short wave because it has a fixed duration, the convolution is non-zero only in a specific part of the signal, according to the translation of the wavelet. Therefore at one level, the wavelet transform accounts for local characteristics of the shape, and each value is linked to a particular range of the signal.

The discrete wavelet transform is applied in a temporal window that must be large enough to contain at least one heartbeat. In order to deal with bradycardial cases, the window is chosen 360 samples large (using a signal sampled at 128 Hz).

The algorithm calculates the absolute maxima of the transform at each level. Then it finds the local maxima of each level, searching for values that exceed a certain threshold. On each level this threshold is set in relation to the absolute maximum of that level according to a certain ratio. A QRS complex is found when the maxima fit through the three levels of wavelet decomposition.

If the heart beats regularly, the beats are segmented into the well-known shape (P wave - QRS complex - T wave). Rapid changes in heart rate could cause some problems: sudden very high heart rate (tachyarrhythmia) can cause two R peaks to be so near that the P wave of one beat is summed upon the T wave of the preceding beat. Obviously this results in a segmented beat without P wave. Ectopic beats are especially difficult to divide, because they interrupt the normal rhythm. Usually they lack T or P wave, are shorter than normal beats, and occur during the resting period of the heart, while the RR interval of the two normal beats remains the same. Such an occasional beat can be very close to the next beat. The algorithm can recognize the presence of ectopic beats by checking for sudden changes in heart rate. This recognition system is robust and gives good results on thousands of beats with an error of 0.4%.

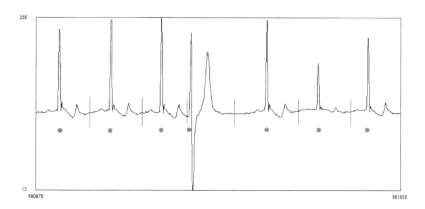

Fig 1: Visual application of the segmentation idea. Heartbeats can be identified by finding their QRS complexes (indicated by dots). Segmentation has to be made after the T waves, as indicated by the lines. Note that the fourth beat is ectopic (ventricular beat without P wave). In this case segmentation has to be made near to its QRS complex

4 Support Vector Approximation of Heartbeat

Using the support vector method in approximating a heartbeat means finding an approximating function f(x)=y; given a set of points $(x_1, y_1), \cdots (x_m, y_m)$. The data are taken from a Holter recording of the ECG signal sampled at 128 samples/sec. The **x** vector corresponds to time values of the individual samples. The **y** vector corresponds to the values of the heart potential

In the heartbeat approximation vectors can be substituted by Gaussian functions

$$k(x_1, x_2) = \frac{1}{\sigma\sqrt{2\pi}} \exp\left(-\frac{(x_1 - x_2)^2}{2\sigma^2}\right), \tag{7}$$

Then the support vector expansion is as follows:

$$f(x) = \sum_{i=1}^{m} (\alpha_i - \alpha_i^*) k(x_i, x) + b \tag{8}$$

The approximating curve can be seen as a sum of a constant b, and *m* Gaussian functions whose width is controlled by σ. Each function is centred at a training point. Increasing the value of σ gives smoother functions. A larger value of σ is needed to have a smooth approximation when the insensitive tube is thick.

In the heartbeat the QRS complex represents the high frequency components. Using a very large σ, the high and narrow complexes cannot be approximated, while using smaller but still too large σ results in an overshoot disturbing strongly the approximation of the Q and S wave. A default value of $\sigma^2=0.4$ gives good results in approximation and low overshoot and ringing.

Once the right value of σ is found, this parameter does not have to be modified and cannot be a source of instability or fault results.

In order to get more accurate, but at the same time noise-free approximation, the value of σ can be made to vary locally, according to some *a priori* knowledge about the frequency contents of the signal and their localisation. Using varying values of σ means using a tube with varying elasticity:

In approximating the heartbeat, two values of σ^2 were used. The value for the QRS complex, represented by 7 samples is 0.3. For the rest of the signal the value $\sigma^2=1.5$ gives much better results in smoothness. The result is a perfect approximation of the QRS complex and a smooth approximation of the P and T waves.

The high frequencies are present only in the QRS complex. The position of the QRS complex within the vector of samples is written in the header that precedes the vector of samples. The SVM (its implementation in C++) can then use this value to initialize the different values of σ^2.

The support vector algorithm builds an approximation of a function using training points that are important for the approximation and that have corresponding Lagrange multipliers different than zero (and smaller than C). The irrelevant points for the approximation have zero Lagrange multipliers and do not contribute to the calculation of the support vector expansion. Thus, the approximating function is built using a subset of the original training set. Furthermore the Lagrange multipliers represent the importance the individual training points have in the approximation. But even those Lagrange multipliers that are equal to zero contain an implicit information about the position of the corresponding component in time domain.

The width of insensitive tube allows a large range of modifications in the algorithm. It modifies the distance of the approximating function with respect to the approximated function at the training points. In approximating the heartbeats with a uniform σ, the value of ε chosen is ε = 0.1. The larger ε, the more the approximating shape resembles a baseline with some "bumps" upon it.

In the approximation of heartbeats, the value of C allows clipping of the multiplier values, providing an upper limit for them. The value of C is set to 1000.

Applying varying values of σ as described above allows using a larger value of ε. Its default was set to 2.5. This value gives a small relative error on QRS complexes. In the approximation of P and T waves the use of a larger value of σ^2 allows a smooth representation with a larger tube. The larger value of ε allows to decrease the number of support vectors in these waves.

The calculated Lagrange multipliers are used for signal parameterisation.

QRS complex has width greater than 0.11 s. At a sampling rate of 64 samples/s this corresponds to maximum 7 samples or 7 parameters of the SVM regression;

For a normal heart rate the PR interval remains the same: approximately 0.18 s or 11 samples. The PQ interval is characterised by 7 samples. These 7 parameters allow parameterisation of the P wave in the most general cases. When studying atrial fibrillation, where the P wave is substituted by a series of F waves, it could be necessary to approximate a longer part of the signal, taking 20 parameters. The normal beat is too short to take 20 parameters of the P wave. In this case these lacking parameters are taken equal to the lowest, negative parameter preceding the P wave. It corresponds to simulating a short resting period preceding the P wave.

The QT interval is at maximum 0.34 s long, i.e. 23 samples. This means that from the end of the S wave until the end of the T wave there are approximately 16 parameters. Hence, each heartbeat is represented by 30 parameters – Lagrange multipliers of support vector approximation.

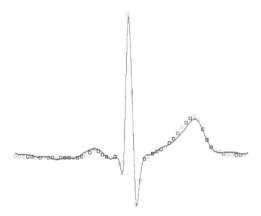

Fig 2: Smooth approximation of a heartbeat showing the data set: red circles are support vectors, black rectangles are the points not involved in the approximation.

5 Support Vector Classification

Classification consists of two steps: training and testing [1, 2, 3, 6]. The training starts up with creation of the training set. Patterns representing classes should be carefully chosen by physicians. E.g., if we want to separate normal heartbeats from ones related to myocardial infarction, we must choose a training set that is complete of all possible shapes of heartbeats that indicate a myocardial infarction. Hence, it is evident that quality of this set decides on the success of the training phase. Below we present some results of SVM classifier score. The result of training is a set of Lagrange multipliers of the dual problem solved by SVM classifier. When we obtain alphas for two classes, we do not need to generate them anymore, they are enough for any test data, and they can separate only the two classes which SVM has been trained by. The Lagrange multipliers determine the position of the separating hyperplane in a space of at most 30 dimensions; depending on shapes to be separate. Hence, we are able to classify patterns whose target is unknown. Output results are produced by SVM theory. When we need to classify more than 2 classes an SVM tree has to be used.

Sometimes we attempt to separate shapes whose differences are related to higher frequencies components and sometimes with lower ones. Typically higher frequencies are differences in QRS complexes, which are more evident; hence there is a large variation among alpha values. In this case, SVM classifier separates patterns considering parameters describing QRS complexes as the most significant ones and other differences in the other part of the signal are not significant for classification. It is an advantage when we do not want to consider variations in P and T waves when we are looking for modifications in QRS complexes but there is also a drawback. If we are interested in variations of lower frequencies, the details of high frequencies components may be ignored. For this reason, we decided to perform training not always with all the parameters representing the entire compressed approximation of each heartbeat, but to use only parameters corresponding to selected parts of the heartbeat.

6 Results of Shape Recognition

In order to illustrate the usefulness of our approach we have selected 7 case studies. The calculations proceeded as follows: some pathological and normal beats were chosen from the patient's Holter recording with the help of cardiologists. The learning sets composed of heartbeats indicated and classified by cardiologists consisted of 7 to 17 examples. The beats were segmented, approximated and parameters were calculated and selected with respect to the pathologies. The classifier was trained giving rise to a certain number of support vectors. The low number of support vectors (2 to 6) with respect to the total number of beats in the training file states the efficiency of heartbeat shape representation.

The segmentation of whole Holter records was obtained in some minutes with an error smaller than 0.15%. Segmented records were parameterized with respect to the parameters chosen for that case and classified using a trained machine. The classification succeeded with an error smaller than 0,3% showing thus good generalisation. This score is valid both on false alarms and false positives, i.e. no more than 0.3 % of pathological beats classified as normal and no more than the same 0.3 % of normal classified as pathological.

In details, the following results were obtained:
- Diagnosis made on patient N3 revealed the presence of ectopic beats which have alterations in the QRS complex with respect to the normal beat (fig 3). The segmented beats were approximated producing 7 parameters of the QRS complex. The classifier distinguished pathological from normal beats with 0.1% error calculated on the Holter record of approximately 90 000 beats.
- Patient MIO4 has pathological beats with alterations in the S and T waves with respect to the normal beat. The segmented beats were approximated producing parameters of QRS+T, or only T wave. The classifier distinguished pathological from normal beats with 0.3% error calculated on an entire Holter record.

- Patient N17 has pathological beats with alterations in the P and T waves with respect to the normal beat. The segmented beats were approximated producing 20 parameters of the P wave and the fixed 16 of T wave. The classifier distinguished pathological from normal beats with 0.1% error calculated on an entire Holter record.
- Patient N105 has two kind of pathological beats (fig 4), both with alterations in the QRS complex and T wave with respect to the normal beat. The segmented beats were approximated producing parameters of QRS complex and T wave, or of T wave only. Classification was made, first distinguishing only one type of pathological beat. Then, an SVM tree was made classifying normal beats and two kind of pathological beats into three classes. Both classifications succeeded with 0.1% error.
- Patient N11 has pathological beats with alterations in the R, S and T waves with respect to the normal beat. The segmented beats were approximated producing parameters of the QRS complex and T wave, or of T wave only. The classifier was trained with the training file of patient N105. It distinguished patient N11 pathological beats from normal beats with 1% error calculated on an entire Holter record.
- Patient K4 has paroxymal atrial fibrillation with alterations in the P wave with respect to the normal beat. In this case the P wave is substituted by a series of small F waves. The segmented beats were approximated producing 20 parameters of the P wave. The classifier distinguished pathological from normal beats with 0.1% error calculated on a subset of beats.
- Patient N87, as patient K4 has pathological beats with alterations in the P wave with respect to the normal beat. The segmented beats were approximated producing 20 parameters of the P wave. The classifier distinguished pathological from normal beats with 0.1% error calculated on a subset of beats.

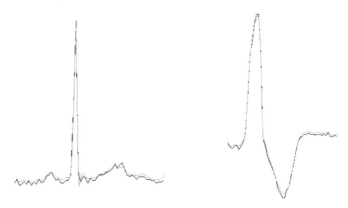

Fig. 3. Patient N3 normal and pathological heartbeats.

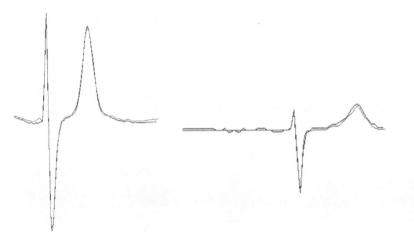

Fig. 4. Patient N105 Supraventricular and premature ventricular heartbeats.

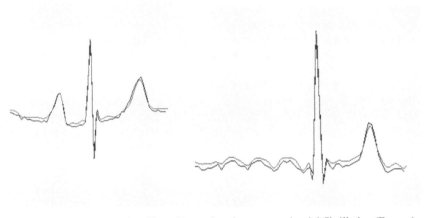

Fig. 5. Patient K4 normal and beat (P wave) and paroxyzmal atrial fibrillation (F wave).

7 Conclusions

Our system is a supervised learning machine. The input patterns are heartbeats, each represented by m parameters. Each point has a label that corresponds to a type of pathology or at least to some precise features within the beat shape. After the learning phase, the machine becomes able to find the labels of new points by comparing them with those it was trained on, or, more precisely, by exploiting the knowledge gathered from the training set. The machine becomes able to make a classification of points.

Actually, we performed different parameterisation for each analysed heartbeat. Since the SVM classifiers are probabilistic by nature, the discrimination of shapes represented by our parameterisation algorithm is consistent and statistically robust.

In the case of binary classification the support vector machine finds the optimal separating hyperplane between two classes. This hyperplane is determined by the support vectors - the training points that are nearest to the boundary between the classes. Their number with respect to the number of points in the training file indicates the difficulty in separating the classes

SVM was trained with a series of heartbeats selected and commented by cardiologists participating in this research. Then the machine performed classification of thousands of beats taken from the Holter records with surprising results.

A well-trained machine can classify heartbeats according to their shape with low error rate. Apart from classifying beats according to the shape of QRS complexes, the machine can also recognise differences in the lower frequency content of the beat, e.g. in P and T waves or ST segment. Experiments on patients affected by paroxymal atrial fibrillation gave excellent results. Pathological beats with small series of F waves substituting the P wave, were identified with very low error

These results pave the way to detection of important alterations in heart functionality and preventing fatal diseases for human beings, by automatic analysis.

We plan to compare our results with another methods on large, well-known data set, as e.g. Physionet database.

Acknowledgments: Work supported by Dean of the Faculty of Electronics and Information Technology, Warsaw University of Technology and partially supported by SOCRATES program. J. Tijink and G. Vumbaca were supported by "La Sapienza" University scholarship. We thank Prof. Dr. Med. G. Opolski for critical remarks.

References

[1] V. N. Vapnik *Statistical Learning Theory*, Wiley, New York, 1998.
[2] B. Schölkopf, C. J. C. Burges and A. J. Smola (eds.): *Advances in Kernel Methods - Support Vector Learning*, MIT Press, 1999
[3] N. Cristianini, J. Shaw-Taylor: *Support Vector Machines*, Cambridge University Press, 2000
[4] J. Platt: *Sequential Minimal Optimization: A fast algorithm for training support vector machines*, Tech. Rep. MSR-TR-98-14, Microsoft Research, 1998
[5] J. Millet-Roig, R. Ventura-Galiano, F. J. Chorro-Gasco, A. Cebrian; Support Vector Machine for Arrhythmia Discrimination with Wavelet-Transform-Based Feature Selection, *Computers in Cardiology* 2000, 27, pp. 407-410
[6] L. Devroye, L. Györfi, G. Lugosi: *A Probabilistic Theory of Pattern Recognition*, Springer-Verlag, New York Berlin Heidelberg 1996

Monitoring of Sleep Apnea in Children Using Pulse Transit Time

Jacopo Pagani[1], Maria Pia Villa[1], Giovanni Calcagnini[2], Enrica Lombardozzi[1], Federica Censi[2], Samantha Poli[2,3], Pietro Bartolini[2], Vincenzo Barbaro[2], Roberto Ronchetti[1]

1 Department of Pediatrics; II Faculty S. Andrea University of Rome "La Sapienza"
2 Biomedical Engineering Laboratory, Istituto Superiore di Sanità, Viale Regina Elena 299, 00161 Roma, Italy
{Barbaro, Bartolin, Giovanni.Calcagnini, Censi}@iss.it
3 Department of Information and System Science, University of Rome, Italy
poli@dis.uniroma1.it

Abstract. Aim of this study was to validate the use of pulse transit time (PTT) as a method to monitor sleep apnea in children. PTT was estimated as the interval between between the ECG R-wave and the point at which the pulse wave at the finger reached 90% amplitude. First, we assessed changes in the PTT during breathing against known resistances in 15 awake children; resistance was applied with a modified nose and mouth two-way non rebreathing face mask, having the inhalation valve port fitted with drilled plastic cylinders. Second, we analyzed 20 events of obstructive apnea and 90 events of central apnea during sleep in 10 children. Our data showed a good correlation between the inspiratory effort and the PTT oscillations amplitude. In addition PTT oscillations amplitude tuned out to successfully discriminate central from obstructive apnea.

1. Introduction

Monitoring of respiratory effort during sleep plays an important role in polysomnographic studies, since increased upper airway resistance causes sleep fragmentation and daytime symptoms [1-3]. Respiratory effort is usually assessed by measuring changes in endoesophageal pressure (Pes) through an endoesophageal balloon catheter [4]. This technique has several disadvantages: first it causes some discomfort and can lead to fragmentary sleep [5][6]; second, the presence of the esophageal monitor can alter the normal respiratory pattern in children during sleep [7]. Recently a noninvasive method for measuring respiratory effort has been proposed. It is based on the estimation of the pulse transit time (PTT), the time needed for the pulse wave to travel from the aortic valve to the periphery, estimated as the delay between the R-wave in the ECG and the arrival of the pulse wave at the finger as determined by pulse oxymetry [8]. It has been demontrated that PTT oscillations yield a valid measure of inspiratory effort: a significant correlation of oscillations in endoesophageal pressure - induced by an episode of augmented airways resistance - and PTT oscillations between inspiration and expiration has been found in adults with

A. Colosimo et al. (Eds.): ISMDA 2002, LNCS 2526, pp. 144-150, 2002.

obstructive sleep apnea syndrome [9]. From a physiological point of view, the PTT discloses acute changes in arterial pressure generated by increased oscillations in pleural pressure due to inspiratory effort induced by obstructive events.

These observations support PTT as an alternative to esophageal pressure measurement for quantitatively assessing inspiratory efforts in adults [10]. What is now lacking are data on the use of PTT in children. Our aim in this study was to validate the usefulness of PTT as a method for monitoring sleep apnea in children.

2. Methodology

2.1 Experimental Protocols

In the first protocol we assessed changes in PTT during breathing against known resistances in 15 awake children (age range 5 to 12 years; mean age 8.3 ± 2.74, 9 boys). The children were selected among patients attending our pediatric service for routine assessment. Participants were tested in the supine position. Each child was fitted with a custom designed nasal and mouth two-way non rebreathing face mask (Series 7910 - Hans Rudolph Inc, Kansas City, Missouri - USA) modified to simulate an inspiratory effort. The inhalation valve port of the mask was adapted to lodge three small plastic cylinders (inner diameter 3, 5 and 8 mm). The openings were gauged to obtain respiratory resistances of 0.064 – 0.010 – and 0.008 mmHg/ml/sec for inspiratory flows ranging from 50 to 250 ml/sec. No extra respiratory resistance was applied to the expiratory port. The mask was also equipped with a transducer for measuring negative pressure generated by inspiratory efforts (Figure 1).

After a 3-min trial to stabilize breathing at zero resistance (baseline), the three progressive resistance levels were applied to the inspiratory port, allowing 3 minutes for each trial and a 2-min recovery period with zero resistance between each trial. Subjects were asked to breathe normally through the nose, to relax and to remain still during measurement. Before starting the protocol, all the children received a short training session. To make sure that sequence had no effect on measurements resistances were applied in random order.

In the second protocol, we analyzed episodes of either central or obstructive apnoeas from 10 children undergoing complete polysomnografic investigation. The episodes were selected by a trained operator by manual scoring of oronasal, thoracic and abdominal traces.

In both protocols, the physiological variables were recorded with a Grass multi-channel instrument (Model Heritage Grass Instruments, Quincy, Mass, USA) and sampled at 250 Hz. Polygraphic data included electrocardiogram (II Lead); arterial blood oxyhemoglobin saturation (SaO_2) and pulse-wave (PW) recorded with a pulse oximeter (NELCOR NPB290) at the finger, mask pressure (only for the first protocol), and abdominal and chest movements (by inductive plethysmography). In the full polysomnographic recordings (second protocol), oronasal flow, abdominal and chest movements, EEG and EOG were also recorded.

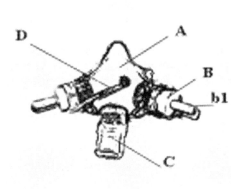

Figure 1. (A) Face mask. (B) The inhalation valve port (B), adapted to lodge small plastic cylinders (b1). (C) The expiratory port with no extra respiratory resistance. (D) Transducer for measuring negative pressure generated by inspiratory efforts.

2.2 PTT Estimation

Data were digitally acquired and transferred to a personal computer. PTT was calculated with a software custom designed in our laboratory. R-waves were detected according to the methods of Pan and Tompkins [11]. Parabolic interpolation of QRS was used to refine the R-wave detection. After the R-wave had been detected the relative minimum and maximum PW were identified in the same beat. PTT was calculated as the interval between the ECG R-wave and the point at which the PW reached 90% amplitude (PW maximum – PW minimum).

We also calculated the amplitude of PTT oscillations (ΔPTT) as suggested by Pitson et al. [12]. The ΔPTT was calculated as the difference between the maximum and minimum PTT values within the same respiratory cycle.

The maximum and minimum PTT were detected manually for every respiratory cycle. For each breathing cycle we also measured the maximal intra-mask pressure drop (Pdrop). For each subject we analyzed 16 consecutive breaths from the second and third minute of each 3-min breathing trial at baseline and against resistance. We calculated the average ΔPTT and Pdrop over 16 consecutive breaths, for each resistance.

3. Results

Of the 15 participants selected for the first protocol, 13 children completed the trial and two failed to do so because of poor compliance with the procedure.

The various resistances applied left the mean, maximum and minimum PTT values substantially unchanged. As the applied inspiratory resistance increased, the mean

ΔPTT increased significantly (from 11.13 ± 1.41 at zero resistance to 21.02 ± 3.10 at maximum; ANOVA Friedman p <0.05; figure 2).

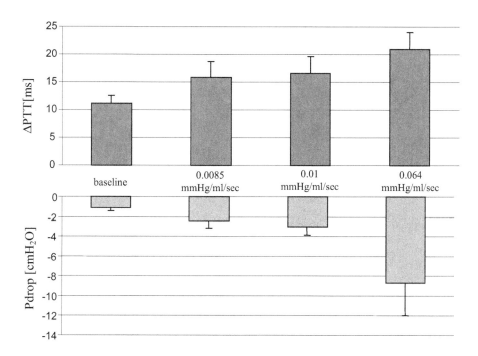

Figure 2. ΔPTT (top) and Pdrop (bottom) averaged all over the population during baseline, and during the application of the inspiratory resistances (0.0085, 0.01, and 0.064mm Hg/ml/sec).

A positive logarithmic correlation was found (R^2 = 0.544) between Pdrop values and ΔPTT values (Figure 3).

From the polysomnographic data of the 10 children analyzed during sleep, we extracted 20 events of obstructive apnea and 90 events of central apnea. We found that mean PTT values do not significantly changed between central and obtructive apnea, while ΔPTT values during obstrutive apnea was significantly higher that that obtained from central apnea (p<0.001,Mann-Whitney U-test for unpair data; figure 4).

4. Discussion

The results obtained in this study indicate that PTT is a sensitive descriptor of inspiratory effort in awake children, and thus represents a valid noninvasive alternative to the endoesophageal balloon technique for measuring inspiratory effort. Our data show a good correlation between the induced inspiratory effort and ΔPTT values. Slight pressure falls in the mask (-8.31 ± 3.35 cmH$_2$O) induced important

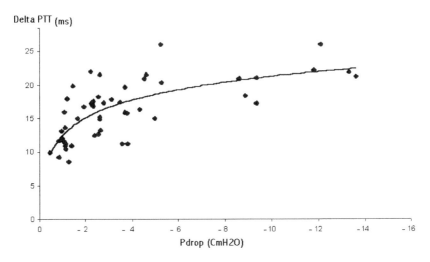

Figure 3. Positive logarithmic correlation ($R^2 = 0.544$) between Pdrop values and ΔPTT values.

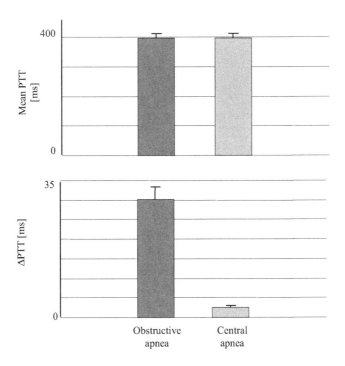

Figure 4. Mean PTT (top) and ΔPTT values obteined during obstructive (dark grey) and central (light grey) episodes, averaged all over the analyzed events.

changes in mean ΔPTT values from baseline (11.13 ± 1.41 vs 21.02 ± 3; $p< 0.001$). ΔPTT also increased significantly already at a Pdrop of about -1 cm H_2O (Pdrop from -1.10 ± 0.31 to -2.42 ± 0.75 cm H_2O; $p <0.001$ - ΔPTT from 11.13 ± 1.41 to 15.82 ± 2.90; $p<0.001$). This finding shows that ΔPTT is a sensitive indicator capable of describing even small changes in inspiratory effort.

Another interesting finding is that as the pressure exerted on the respiratory airways increased, ΔPTT increased not linearly but in a logarithmic manner thus tending to saturate. This behavior may have arisen from several cardiovascular factors, mostly unknown, such as elasticity and compliance of the arterial vascular tree. These factors may prevent the pulse-wave transit velocity from increasing or slowing down beyond a certain limit.

We also found that ΔPTT values are capable to discriminate central from obstructive apnea. This latter result is consistent with the different mechanisms involved in central and obstructive apneas: in central apnoeas, no stimulus to the respiratory muscles is generated and no changes in pleural pressure occur. Conversely, obstructive apneas cause large swings in pleural pressure, producing oscillations in blood pressure detected by PTT. This finding suggests that ΔPTT measurement could have a clinical application also in polysomnographic studies to monitor sleep apnea in children, helping in simplifying portable polysomnographic systems.

References

1. Guilleminault C, Pelayo R, Leger D, Clerk A, Bocian RC. Validation of the sleep-EVAL system against clinical assessments of sleep disorders and polysomnographic data. Sleep 1999;22(7):925-930.
2. Guilleminault C, Stoohs R, Clerk A, Simmons J, Labanowski M. From obstructive sleep apnea syndrome to upper airway resistance syndrome: consistency of daytime sleepiness. Sleep 1992;15(6 Suppl):S13-S16
3. Guilleminault C, Stoohs R, Clerk A, Cetel M, Maistros P. A cause of excessive daytime sleepiness. The upper airway resistance syndrome. Chest 1993;104(3):781-787.
4. Baydur A, Behrakis PK, Zin WA, Jaeger M, Milic-Emili J. A simple method for assessing the validity of the esophageal balloon technique. Am Rev Respir Dis. 1982;126(5):788-791.
5. Hoffstein V Snoring Chest 1996; 109: 201-222
6. Chediak AD, Demirozu MC, Nay KN. Alpha EEG sleep produced by balloon catheterization of the esophagus. Sleep 1990;13(4): 369-370.
7. Woodson BT, Wooten MR. A multisensor solid-state pressure manometer to identify the level of collapse in obstructive sleep apnea. Otolaryngol Head Neck Surg. 1992;107(5):651-656.
8. Smith RP, Argod J, Pepin JL, Levy PA. Pulse transit time: an appraisal of potential clinical applications. Thorax. 1999;54(5):452-457.
9. Pitson DJ, Sandell A, van de Hoot R, Stradling JR. Pulse transit time as a measure of respiratory effort in patient with obstructive sleep apnoea Eur Resp J 1995;8:1669-1674

10. Pitson DJ, Sandell A, van den Hout R, Stradling JR. Use of pulse transit time as a measure of inspiratory effort in patients with obstructive sleep apnoea. Eur Respir J. 1995;8(10):1669-1674.
11. Pan J, Tompkins WJ A real-time QRS detection algorithm. IEEE Trans Biomed Eng 1985; 32(3):230-236.
12. Pitson DJ, Chhina N, Knijn S, van Herwaaden M, Stradling J. Changes in pulse transit time and pulse rate as a markers of arousal from sleep in normal subjects. Clinical Science 1994; 87:269-273

Linear and Nonlinear Evaluation of Ventricular Arrhythmias

Joseph P. Zbilut[1], Peter A. Santucci[2], Shiow-Ying Yang[3], and
Janice L. Podolski[4]

[1] Dept. of Molecular Biophysics and Physiology, Rush Medical College
1653 W. Congress, Chicago, IL 60612 USA
Joseph_P_Zbilut@rush.edu
[2] Section of Cardiology, Rush Medical College
1653 W. Congress, Chicago, IL 60612 USA
psantucc@rush.edu
[3] National Taiwan University, No.1, Section 4
Tapei, Taiwan, Republic of China
[4] Dept. of Pharmacology, Rush Medical College
1653 W. Congress, Chicago, IL 60612 USA

Abstract. Ventricular arrhythmias are often difficult to evaluate on a
quantitative basis. We present here the results of analysis with traditional
Fourier transforms, and recurrence quantification analysis. The results
indicate that recurrence quantification can better distinguish them, most
likely due to its ability to handle nonstationary, nonlinear data.

1   Introduction

Ventricular arrhythmias are potentially lethal and include monomorphic ventricular tachycardia (MVT), polymorphic ventricular tachicardia (PMVT), and
ventricular fibrillation (VF). Although these arrhythmias can be usually distinguished by inspection of the surface electrocardiogram (ECG), at times, this may
be difficult. Additionally, the increased use of automatic devices necessitates reliable means of analyzing ventricular rhythms independent of human inspection.

Generally, descriptions of these arrhythmias has been in the form of qualitative features and rates. Some attempts have used fast Fourier transforms (FFT),
however, results can be confounding due to the mathematical assumptions of
the FFT; namely, stationarity, and relatively long data length [1]. These issues
are complicated by the fact that the surface ECG is an empirical phenomenon
whose various leads provide, at times, differing profiles. It has also been pointed
out that these arrhythmias are nonlinear, whose determinism is often hidden by
the supposed "chaotic" nature of their surface ECG representation.

We present here the results from an attempt to compare FFT analysis of
these arrhythmias with their recurrence quantification (RQA) analysis. RQA is
a technique which simply quantifies recurrences (patterns) without prior transformation as is the case with FFTs.

A. Colosimo et al. (Eds.): ISMDA 2002, LNCS 2526, pp. 151–157, 2002.

2   Recurrences

Recurrences have had a long history. Poincaré is perhaps the most famous for describing them in the context of dynamical systems as points which visit a small region of phase space. Also, the statistical literature points out that recurrences are the most basic of relations [2]. In this respect, it is important to reiterate the fact that calculation of recurrence times, unlike other methods such as FFTs, Wigner-Ville or wavelets, requires no transformation of the data, and can be used for both linear and nonlinear systems. Because recurrences are simply tallies, they make no mathematical assumptions. Given a reference point, $\mathbf{X}_0$, and a ball of radius r, a point is said to recur if $B_r(\mathbf{X}_0) = \{\mathbf{X} : \| \mathbf{X} - \mathbf{X}_0 \| \leq r\}$. A trajectory of size N falling within $B_r(\mathbf{X}_0)$ is denoted as $S_1 = \{\mathbf{X}_{t_1}, \mathbf{X}_{t_2}, ..., \mathbf{X}_{t_i}...\}$ with the recurrence times defined as $T_1(i) = t_{i+1} - t_i, i = 1, 2, ...N$.

2.1   Recurrence Plots

Given a scalar time series $\{x(i) = 1, 2, 3, ...\}$ an embedding procedure will form a vector, $\mathbf{X}_i = (x(i), x(i+L), ..., x(i+(m-1)L))$ with m the embedding dimension and L the lag. $\{\mathbf{X}_i = 1, 2, 3, ..., N\}$ then represents the multidimensional process of the time series as a trajectory in m-dimensional space. Recurrence plots (RP) are symmetrical $N \times N$ arrays in which a point is placed at (i, j) whenever a point $\mathbf{X}_i$ on the trajectory is close to another point $\mathbf{X}_j$, as defined by: $\| \mathbf{X}_i - \mathbf{X}_j \| \leq r$ where r is a fixed radius. If the distance falls within this radius, the two vectors are considered to be recurrent, and graphically this can be indicated by a dot. An important feature of such matrixes is the existence of short line segments parallel to the main diagonal, which are deterministic. The absence of such patterns suggest randomness [3].

Unfortunately, beyond general impressions of drift and determinism, the plots of themselves provide no quantification. As a result, RQA was developed to quantify features of such plots [4],[5]. Quantification of recurrences leads to the generation of five variables including: %REC (percent of plot filled with recurrent points); %DET (percent of recurrent points forming diagonal lines, with a minimum of two adjacent points); ENT (Shannon information entropy of the line length distribution); MAXLINE, length of longest line segment (the reciprocal of which is an approximation of the largest positive Liapunov exponent; and is a measure of system divergence); and TREND (measure of the paling of recurrent points away from the central diagonal). These five recurrence variables quantify the deterministic structure and complexity of the plot. In order to follow changes of these variables in time, a "windowed" version of RQA can be performed. Analogous to cross power spectral analysis, cross recurrence analysis is also possible. The data obtained can also be used to obtain estimations of local Liapunov exponents, information entropy, or simply plotted as $N_{recurrences}$ vs. period; i.e., a histogram of recurrence times. In the case of histograms, strictly periodic points demonstrate instrumentally sharp peaks; whereas chaotic or nonlinear systems reveal more or less wider peaks depending upon the radius chosen and noise effects.

2.2   Determining Parameters for Nonstationary Series

As has been emphasized, RQA is useful for understanding nonstationary time series. Yet, since a given system may be changing state; i.e., the relevant degrees of freedom may change, the choice of m, L and r can become confounding. Unfortunately, most algorithms for such choices are based upon computer simulations of well-known, stationary examples. Typically, however, biological systems are rarely stationary, and often exhibit rather sudden changes of state. Nonetheless, some guidelines can be established, based upon available research, and a careful consideration of the import of nonstationarity. (For this and subsequent parameter settings, see [6] for additional discussion.)

Choice of Embedding In the context of nonstationarity, the notion of a "correct" embedding or delay is inappropriate [7]. Instead it becomes important to remember that a sufficiently large embedding be chosen which will "contain" the relevant dynamics (as it may change from one dimensionality to another) as well as account for the effects of noise, which tend to inflate dimension.

Choice of Lag Choice of lag is governed by similar considerations. As a system changes from one dimension to another the effects of the lag are perforce changed. Thus, a so-called "optimal" lag in one embedding, becomes less so as the relevant dimension changes. Although there have been numerous proposals for choice of lag, chief among them the first local minimum of the autocorrelation or mutual information, they all are presented with the assumption of stationarity.

Choice of Radius The object of RQA is to view the recurrences in a locally defined (linear) region of phase space. Practically speaking, however, because of intrinsic and extrinsic noise, too small a value of r results in quantification of the noise only; whereas too large a value captures values which can no longer be considered recurrent. To get to the dynamics proper, a strategy is to calculate %REC for several increasing values of r and to plot the results on a log-log plot to determine a "scaling" region; i.e., where the dynamics are found.

If the data are extremely nonstationary, a scaling region may not be found. The guide then is the %REC. A critical factor is that there be sufficient numbers of recurrences so as to make sense for computation of the other variables. A value of 1% recurrence tends to fulfill this criterion.

3   Materials and Methods

Surface ECGs were obtained from subjects undergoing arrhythmia evaluation in an electrophysiology laboratory. A convenience sample of 14 from each category (MVT, PMVT, VF) were identified. Samples were recorded via the Prucka 4.1 electrophysiologic recorder, digitized at 1000 Hz. Actual analysis was performed on standard leads I, aVF, and V1 to obtain a quasi-orthogonal frame of reference with respect to the chest cavity. A high-pass Butterworth filter (bi-directional) was employed to remove baseline drift. Each exemplar was 2048 points in length (approximately 2 seconds).

Each lead was then subjected to a 2048 point FFT. Dominant frequency (Df), amplitude of dominant frequency (Amp), center frequency (weighted average of frequencies), and half-width of half-height (hwhh) were then calculated. Additionally, the Euclidean norm of the three leads was calculated and subjected to the same analysis. The normed data was then processed by RQA to obtain %REC, %DET, ENT, MAXLINE, and TREND. An embedding of 10, delay of 8 and radius of 5 was used with unit interval normalization (Fig. 1). Also a histogram of recurrence intervals was obtained, to identify significant peaks, their amplitudes, and standard deviations (Fig. 2). To determine which methods better distinguished the arrhythmias, the measured variables were submitted to logistic regression. Significance was set at $p < 0.05$.

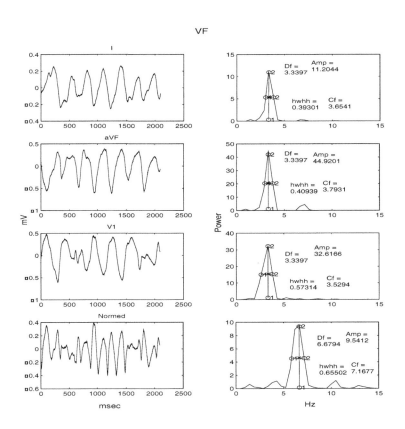

Fig. 1. Calculation of FFT parameters. Time series of leads (left); resultant calculations of respective FFTs (right)

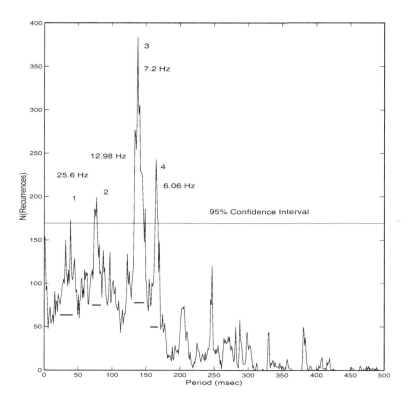

Fig. 2. Recurrence histograms. Confidence intervals (95%) were calculated for the series and peaks exceeding this value were considered significant. Note that only peak no. 3 is equaivalent to that of the power spectrum finding. The other peaks clearly contribute to the lack of definition of the normed series as seen in Fig. 1. Bars below the peaks indicate approx. width of area used to calculate the standard deviation for the peak. This was done through simple inspection

4   Results

The logistic regression procedure demonstrated the superiority of the RQA variables in terms of discriminating the three ventricular arrhythmias (Tables 1 and 2). Additionally, a Kruskal-Wallis test of the standard deviations of the 4th peak of the recurrence histogram peaks was especially prominent in distinguishing VF ($p = 0.036$).

Table 1. Logistic regression results for RQA, Recurrence histogram, and FFT in discriminating between MVT, PVT and VF. Note that although RQA and Rec. Histogram both obtain a $p < 0.001$, the R-squared value for Rec. Histogram is slightly higher than RQA.

Method	R-squared	Chi-square	Significance
Rec. Histogram	0.889	92.983	$p < 0.001$
RQA	0.885	90.897	$p < 0.001$
FFT	0.530	68.882	$p = NS$

Table 2. Classification matrix based on logistic discriminant function. Observed (columns) vs. predicted (rows).

Method		MVT	PVT	VF	%Correct
Rec. Hist.	MVT	14	0	0	100
	PVT	0	14	0	100
	VF	0	0	14	100
	Total %	33.3	33.3	33.3	100
RQA	MVT	13	1	0	92.9
	PVT	0	14	0	100
	VF	0	0	14	100
	Total %	31	35.7	33.3	97.6
FFT	MVT	10	1	3	88.2
	PVT	2	12	0	90.3
	VF	0	0	14	100
	Total %	30.9	31	38.1	90.5

5   Discussion and Conclusion

Inspection of the time series and FFTs of a typical ventricular arrhythmias clearly demonstrates the difficulties encountered in using FFTs with such data. Although one or several leads may demonstrate a dominant frequency, it is not uncommon that one of the three leads show less than instrumental peaks. Additionally, when viewed from the normed lead, the situation becomes more confounding. However, given the nonstationary nature of the signal, and the high likelihood that the signal is also nonlinear, makes an FFT analysis less than optimal [8]. RQA, on the other hand has none of the FFT mathematical requisites. For this reason, it is probable that RQA can provide a clearer picture. This may be especially important for understanding of the temporal variation of ventricular fibrillation, and consequently, the most efficient way of terminating it [9].

References

1. Clayton, R.H., Murray, A.: Linear and Non-linear Analysis of the Surface Electro-cardiogram during Human Ventricular Fibrillation Shows Evidence of Order in the Underlying Mechanism. Med. Bio. Eng. Comp. **37** (1999) 354–358
2. Feller, W.: An Introduction to Probability Theory and Its Applications, Vol. 1. Wiley, New York (1968)
3. Eckmann, J.-P., Kamphorst, S.O., Ruelle, D.: Recurrence Plots of Dynamical Systems. Europhys. Lett. **4** (1987) 973–977
4. Zbilut, J.P., Webber, Jr. C.: Embeddings and Delays as Derived from Quantification of Recurrence Plots. Phys. Lett. A **171** (1992) 199–203
5. Webber, Jr. C.L., Zbilut, J.P.: Dynamical Assessment of Physiological Systems and States Using Recurrence Plot Strategies. J. Appl. Physiol. **76** (1994) 965–973
6. Zbilut, J.P., Thomasson, N., Webber, Jr. C.L.: Recurrence Quantification Analysis as a Tool for Nonlinear Exploration of Nonstationary Cardiac Signals. Med. Eng. Phys. **24** (2002) 53–60
7. Grassberger, P., Schreiber, T., Schaffrath, C.: Non-linear Time Sequence Analysis. Int. J. Bifurcation and Chaos **1** (1991) 521–547
8. Santucci, P., Zbilut, J.P., Mitra, R.: Detecting Undersensing in Implantable Defibrillators Using Recurrence Analysis. Computers in Cardiology **98**(1998) 261–264
9. Mani, V., Xuejun, W., Wood, M.A., Ellenbogen, K.A., Hsia, P.W.: Variation of Spectral Power Immediately Prior to Spontaneous Onset of Ventricular Tachycardia/Ventricular Fibrillation in Implantable Cardioverter Defibrillator Patients. J. Cardiovascular Electrophysiology. **10** (1998) 1586–1596

Invariant and Subject-Dependent Features of Otoacoustic Emissions

Giovanna Zimatore[1], Alessandro Giuliani[2], Stavros Hatzopoulos[3],
Alessandro Martini[3], and Alfredo Colosimo[1]

[1] Dept. of Human Physiology and Pharmacology and CISB,
Univ. of Rome "La Sapienza", 00185 Rome, Italy
colosimo@caspur.it

[2] Ist. Superiore di Sanità, 00185 Rome, Italy

[3] Center of Bioacoustics, Univ. of Ferrara, Italy

Abstract. Transiently-Evoked Otoacoustic Emissions (TEOAEs) from nine normoacousic subjects have been studied by Recurrence Quantification Analysis (RQA) at different stimulation intensities, and their dynamics characterized as for the content of determinism. The same linear scaling of determinism with the stimulation intensity has been found in a well defined intensity interval and in all subjects. Outside that interval and, in particular, above its upper end, subject-dependent features are clearly visible in the form of different maximal levels of determinism. These observations may open the door to a systematic study of the anatomical and physiological bases of both individual and subject-dependent features in otoacoustic emissions.

1 Introduction

Transiently evoked otoacoustic emissions (TEOAEs) correspond to signals coming from the activity of the outer hair cells of the inner ear responding to an artificially generated acoustic stimulation. These signals are related to the processing of pertinent information by the auditory system and are used both as clinical tools, for detecting hearing impairments, and as probes of the auditory system functioning, for research purposes [1].

The auditory system can be considered as a freely moving dynamical system made coherent by the in-going stimulation, and the induced coherence patterns can be considered the same among different subjects. In this frame, individual differences in stimulus processing might be related to the different deterministic character of the outer hair cells oscillations. In a previous work on TEOAE signals [2] analyzed by recurrence quantification analysis, RQA [3], we demonstrated: i) the close link between the reaching of a given amount of determinism and the correct functionality of the auditory system, and ii) the existence of a marked degree of individuality in normoacousic ears, which produce distinguishable signals in terms of the dynamical features measured by RQA.

A. Colosimo et al. (Eds.): ISMDA 2002, LNCS 2526, pp. 158-166, 2002.
© Springer-Verlag Berlin Heidelberg 2002

In this work we analyze both the invariant and the subject-dependent features of TEOAE responses and show that the former type of features consists in the same linear relation between the increasing intensity of the stimuli and the increasing determinism of the responses, while the latter type consists in different maximal levels of determinism. These "maximal levels" are shown to correlate with the lowest value of the stimulus intensity at which DET becomes detectable. This could, in principle, help in localize the structural basis of individuality at a pre-cochlear level.

Assuming the auditory system as a flexible, adaptive machinery, the existence of a linear coupling between stimulus intensity and determinism can be also considered as one facet of the complex, physiological mechanisms through which the system self-organizes in response to different incoming stimulations.

2 Materials and Methods

2.1 Data Sets

The TEOAE signals were collected in the Audiology Department (Center of Bioacoustics) of the University of Ferrara – Italy, from the right ears of 9 adult female subjects (age range: 26.8 ± 7.1 years) chosen on the basis of the absence of: i) any pathophysiological objective sign of clinical relevance, and ii) any systematic pharmacological treatment within three months from the acquisition of the TEOAE response. Click-evoked emissions were recorded in a sound-attenuated booth with the subject seating adjacent to the recording equipment, using an ILO 88 system (Otodynamics inc.) with standard adult ILO probes.

2.2 TEOAE Stimulation Protocols

To record the TEOAE responses, click stimuli with a relatively flat acoustic spectrum for frequencies between 0.5-5 kHz were used, according to a non-linear stimulation protocol. The latter included three clicks of positive polarity followed by a fourth click with inverse polarity and intensity equal to the sum of the previous three. For each subject 16 different responses were collected, corresponding to 16 levels of click stimuli ranging from 35dB to 80dB. The responses were high-pass filtered at 500 Hz. Every accepted response was the average of at least 260 individual responses for each subject.

2.3 RQA Parameters

RQA projects the signals into a multidimensional space through the set up of an embedding matrix, having as columns the lagged copies of the original signal by a fixed delay. On this matrix, RQA identifies time correlations that cannot be observed in one dimension. The first step of the analysis is the computation of the Euclidean distance between every row pair in the embedding matrix, in order to work out a distance matrix and visualize it in the form of a recurrence plot. In this plot, each pair of rows whose euclidean distance falls below a user-defined threshold (radius) is considered as recurrent, and the corresponding point is darkened. From here on, the calculation of the quantitative recurrence parameters is straightforward:

REC (% Recurrence) is simply the percentage of recurrent points in the plot; DET (% Determinism) corresponds to the percentage of recurrent points that occur in lines; MAXLINE corresponds to the length of the longest deterministic line; ENT (Entropy) is an entropy computed by the application of the Shannon formalism to the length distribution of deterministic lines; TREND is a stationarity indicator, corresponding to the decrease of recurrent points density farther and farther away from the main diagonal of the recurrence plot.

In this paper we make use of % Recurrence (REC), % Determinism (DET), and Entropy (ENT), calculated with the following choice of parameters: lag (delay in the embedding procedure) = 1; embedding dimension (number of elements in the rows of the embedding matrix) = 10; radius = 15 and line = 8 (for more details see reff. 2, 3). It is worth noting that the radius is expressed as percentage of the mean distance between rows, in order to make variance- and amplitude-independent (and hence only order dependent) the observed dynamical features of the signal.

2.4 Principal Component Analysis (PCA)

Principal Component Analysis (PCA) is a quite common statistical technique [4] whose aim is to project a multivariate data set into a space of orthogonal axes - called principal components – selected, one after the other, on the basis of the maximal variance explained in the space of the original variables. The presence of correlations between the original variables allows for the reduction of dimensionality of the data set in the new space without noticeable loss of information Moreover, since the principal components are by construction orthogonal to each other, this allows a clear separation of the different and independent properties characterizing the data set. In other words, going from the original variables to a principal component space, any statistically significant observation, made on any axis, points to a truly autonomous effect.

3 Results and Discussion

Figure 1 reports the graph of typical TEOAEs taken at very low (panel a) and saturating (panel b) stimulation intensity. In TEOAE clinical studies [5], the responses are often evoked by high intensity stimuli (>65 dB), and the difference between normal and pathological hearing are apparent in terms of the waveform reproducibility. This is indicated by the so called REPRO value, corresponding to an estimate, on a 0-100 scale, of the correlation between two waveforms (A, B) recorded in alternating sampling times. For the 35 dB stimulus the resulting signals are barely distinguishable from the baseline noise and the two A and B waveforms are not super-imposable (REPRO: 4.4 at 35 dB; REPRO: 99.1 at 80 dB). As shown in figure 1, going from very low intensity (panel a) to the saturating phase (panel b) the signal increases both in amplitude and in relative organization: an

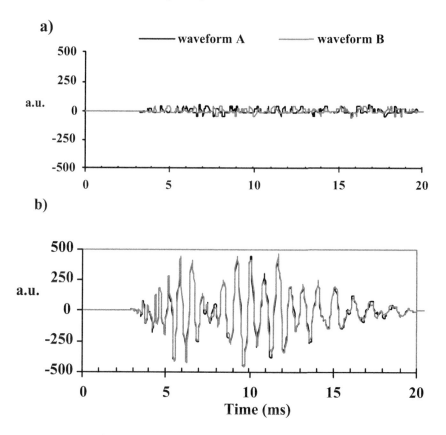

Fig. 1. TEOAE responses at different intensity stimulations. Panels a) and b) contain the two waveforms (A, B) of TEOAE responses evoked by intensities of 35 and 80 dB, respectively. On the time axis, 20.48 ms. correspond to 512 digitized data points

irregular, noisy activity changes into a markedly oscillatory behaviour. It should be noticed that, by virtue of RQA, attention may be exclusively focussed on the variation in the signal ordering upon increasing the stimulation intensity, while changes in variance and amplitude are ruled out.

Figure 2 reports, for all the nine subjects studied in this work, the progressive increase of the deterministic character of TEOAEs as the stimulus intensity increases. This is a demonstration of the external stimulus acting as an order parameter, i.e. introducing a progressive coherence in the activity of the hair outer cells. The increase of DET reaches a plateau, corresponding to the saturation activity of the cochlea.

Three different segments of determinism in the TEOAE can be detected . In figure 2: the first phase (A) corresponds to sub-threshold stimuli, where the outer hair cells are characterized by physiological, spontaneous activities; a second phase (B), characterized by a linear increase in determinism following the stimulus intensity; and a third one (C), an almost constant saturation state, where the system reaches maximal activity.

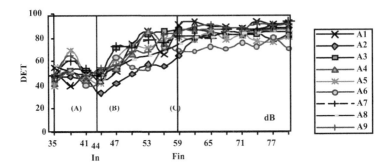

Fig. 2. Deterministic structure of TEOAEs evoked by different stimuli intensities. the initial and final points of the linear phase (B) are marked "In" and "Fin", respectively. (A) and (C) indicate the sub-threshold and saturated phases, respectively

During the A phase the system displays a very noisy activity, while in the C phase it is organized into a quasi-harmonic, extremely ordered state (Fig.1a,b).

If one looks at the linear phase (B), it appears that for all subjects (with the only partial exception of subject A6) a very similar angular coefficient holds, linking the stimulus intensity to the percentage determinism (Table 1). This corresponds to a very similar self-organization dynamics in different individuals, based upon recruiting (and making coherent) subsequent portions of the auditory system.

We know, however, from previous results [3] that in the saturation phase the TEOAEs show a marked individual character and act as a sort of "auditory fingerprint" of single individuals.

Table 1. Linear fitting of DET values for individual responses in the 44 dB –58 dB interval of intensity stimulation

Subject	Linear equation	R square
A1	y = 2.75x – 72.90	0.684
A2	y = 2.04x – 54.41	0.944
A3	y = 2.19x - 37.52	0.847
A4	y = 2.38x - 52.29	0.819
A5	y = 2.25x - 48.30	0.818
A6	y = 1.47x - 16.49	0.585
A7	y = 1.79x - 20.94	0.692
A8	y = 1.65x - 22.85	0.990
A9	y = 2.13x – 40.82	0.948

a)

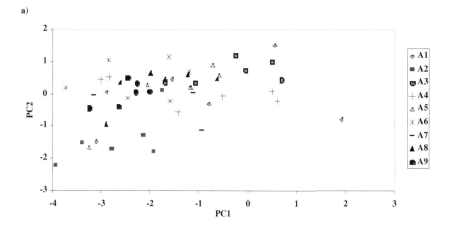

b)

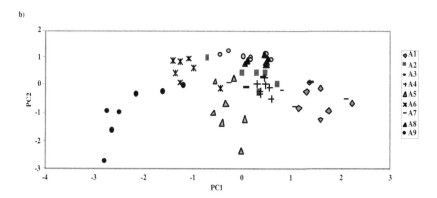

Fig. 3. Clustering of individual TEOAE responses in a PC1/PC2 plane. The same symbol is used for signals recorded, from the same ear of the same subject, in subsequent experimental sessions. Each signal was separately analyzed and plotted in the PC1/PC2 plane obtained from a previous set of measurements (learning set) carried out, under similar conditions [2]. Panels a) and b) refer to signals evoked by intensity stimuli in the linear phase and in the saturation phase, respectively (see figure 2)

In order to contrast the invariance typical of the linear phase (B) with the individual character of the saturation phase (A), we generated, for each phase, the space of the principal components computed on the RQA parameters, where TEOAE signals was described by means of the REC, DET and ENT parameters. The matrix having as rows the signals and as columns the corresponding parameters was subjected to a principal component analysis in order to obtain a component space spanned by orthogonal axes and able to represent in two dimensions (instead of three) most of the dynamical features of the studied signals. Independent analyses were carried out for the B and the C phases, to highlight differences (if any) in the discrimination ability of the two phases. The component space reported in figure 3 reveals that the linear phase does not allow to recognize signals pertaining to the same individual (panel a), while clusters of signals of the same individual clearly appear in the saturation phase (panel b).

The lack of subject-related features in the B phase indicates the same basic scaling of DET in all subjects, and points to the same progressive recruitment of similar structures in the hearing system by stimuli of increasing intensity. This phenomenon could be assimilated, in a way, to the progressive magnetization of paramagnetic materials subjected to a static, magnetic field.

Given the presence in the TEOAEs of all the examined individuals of the same linear scaling of determinism with increasing stimulus intensity, and of a saturated plateau phase displaying a marked individual character, trying to localize the region of this individual character is mandatory. First of all, it is important to check whether this individuality can be evidenced even in the sub-threshold phase, since this would indicate some basic architectural differences of the auditory system, independent of the applied stimulus. A statistical confirmation of the latter statement lies in the significance of the relation existing between the relative positions of different signals in the A phase and in the C phase. This significance was demonstrated by: i) computing all the differences in determinism between any possible couple of subjects both at the initial (In) and at the final (Fin) point of the linear phase in figure 2, corresponding to the low (44 dB) and saturating (59 dB) stimulation intensity, respectively, and ii) checking for the mutual correlation between the corresponding differences (figure 4).

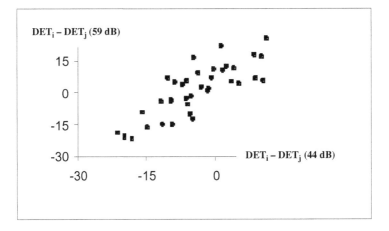

Fig. 4. Correlation between differences in DET of couples of subjects. The two axes represent the differences in DET between each of the 36 (= 9*8/2) possible pairing of of the 9 subjects (i, j) examined in this work, at the beginning (44 dB) and at the end (59 dB) of the linear phase (B) in figure 2

It is easy to realize that the two difference series are highly correlated (r=0.802), pointing to a basic invariance of the mutual location of the different individuals passing from the A to C phase. This means that individual features in the structural organization of the auditory system are equally distinguishable at both the sub-threshold and saturation phases.

4 Conclusions

We observed a progressive increase in coherence of TEOAE signals induced by external stimuli of increasing intensity, which is invariant across different normoacousic subjects. This points to the same general functioning of the system as for the scaling region between stimulus intensity and increase in coherence of the response signal. On the contrary, individual differences clearly appear in terms of the maximal attainable "ordering" in the response, and are correlated with the differences estimated at very low intensity stimulation, below the lower limit of the linear phase.

It is worth to remind that at such low stimulation intensity the REPRO value is of no clinical use, while determinism retains a heuristic power concerning both individuality and, most probably, clinical issues. This is the reason why much of the attention has been dedicated up to now to the saturation phase where, however, the dynamical behaviour of the auditory system cannot be fully explored. Recurrence analysis, due to the high sensitivity to fine dynamical details, allows to focus on previously unexplored portions of the phase space of the system.

If our observations will be confirmed by a more detailed data collection in the critical region around 44 dB stimulation, namely the starting point of the scaling region, a similar origin for the individual features observed in the stationary region and for their common scaling with stimulus intensity could be assessed on a well defined morpho-anatomical basis. To validate this hypothesis, one obvious strategy deals with the analysis of pathological subjects in which the anatomical location of the pathology is known [6-7]. Pathological events (sensorineural hearing loss, otosclerosis...) occurring in different regions (cochlea, middle ear bones, etc.) could be also helpful to identify the origin of the observed dynamical behaviour by means of the same approach used in this work.

An alternative (and complementary) procedure would be to use frequency- instead of intensity-modulated stimuli to identify, if any, different sub-populations of hair cells responding to specific frequencies. In this case, the progressive recruitment of auditory sub-systems observed at increasing stimulus intensities could be reproduced, at the level of the hair cells sub-populations, as an effect of the increasing number of frequencies included in the stimulus.

References

1. Kemp, D. T.,: Stimulated otoacoustic emissions from within the human auditory system. J. Acoust. Soc. Am. **64** (1978) 1386-1391
2. Zimatore, G., Hatzopoulos, S., Giuliani, A., Martini, A., Colosimo, A.: Comparison of transient otoacoustic emission (TEOAE) responses from neonatal and adult ear. J. Appl. Physiol. **92** (2002) 2521-2528
3. Webber, C.L., and Zbilut, J.P.: Dynamical assessment of physiological systems and states using recurrence plot strategy. J. Appl. Physiol. **76** (1994) 965-973
4. Bartholomew, D.J.: The foundation of factor analysis. Biometrika. **71** (1984) 221-2329
5. Hatzopoulos, S., Petruccelli, J., Pelosi, G., Martini, A.: A TEOAE screening protocol based on linear click stimuli: performance and scoring criteria. Acta Otolaryngol. **119**(2) (1999) 135-139

6. Bamiou, D.E., Savy, L., O'Mahoney, C., Phelps, P., Sirimanna, T.,: Unilateral sensorineural hearing loss and its aetiology in childhood: the contribution of computerised tomography in aetiological diagnosis and management. International Journal of Pediatric Otorhinolaryngology. **51** (2) (1999) 91 – 99

7. Qiu, W. W., Yin, S., Stucker, F. J.: Critical evaluation of deafness. Auris Nasus Larynx. **26** (3) (1999) 269 - 276

Short Term Evaluation of Brain Activities in fMRI Data by Spatiotemporal Independent Component Analysis

M. Balsi[1,2], V. Cimagalli[1,2], G. Cruccu[3], G.D. Iannetti[3],
A. Londei[1,2], P.L. Romanelli[1,3]

1. Department of Electronic Engineering, "La Sapienza" University of Rome
via Eudossiana, 18; Rome, Italy I-00184
balsi@uniroma1.it
2. ECONA - Interuniversity Center for Research on Cognitive Processing
in Natural and Artificial Systems; Rome, Italy
3. Department of Neurological Sciences, "La Sapienza" University of Rome
Viale dell'Università, 30; Rome, Italy

Abstract. At present, Independent Components Analysis (ICA) represents the most important and efficient approach for extraction of independent non-Gaussian linearly mixed signals. This statistic-informative technique has been successfully applied to fMRI temporal data, which can be considered as an overlapped mixture of hemodynamic signals, physiological perturbations and noise. In this paper an extension to spatial application of ICA (sICA) was performed. The results confirmed that the spatial approach permits to obtain improved identification of brain activities, even when the temporal length of data is reduced.

1 Introduction

Functional Magnetic Resonance Imaging (fMRI) is becoming a widely used non-invasive tool for disclosing functionally active brain areas in healthy subjects and patients [1]. This technique is based on detection of dynamic responses emerging in the brain in relation to different events–(e.g. somatosensory stimulation, motor performance, cognitive tasks). During neural activation, the regional cerebral blood flow increases, producing a transient local increase of the oxyhaemoglobin: deoxyhaemoglobin ratio. The concurrent increase in signal intensity (the so-called blood oxygen level-dependent effect, BOLD) relies on the magnetization difference between oxy- and deoxyhaemoglobin. Even if the biophysical mechanisms are not fully understood, the signal change is clearly a function of blood flow, volume and oxygenation state [2]. The BOLD contrast is usually measured with T_2^*-weighted gradient recalled EPI (Echo-Planar magnetic resonance Imaging) [3]. Recently this technique has been widely applied to the investigation of pathologies such as epilepsy and brain damages and to research in cognitive processing [4,5]. Because the EPI technique allows capturing one MR image in less than 100 ms, it is possible to iterate the scan, to get a reasonably dense time sampling of brain activity, so that a space-time description of phenomena is available. However, it is to be noted that the

A. Colosimo et al. (Eds.): ISMDA 2002, LNCS 2526, pp. 167-176, 2002.

acquired signal is composed by the experiment-related hemodynamic signals embedded into a large amount of noise due to the sensitivity of the measurement, artifacts caused by small movement of the head, physiological influences as breathing or swallowing, and brain activity not related to the considered stimulus. For these reasons, post-processing of the data set is mandatory. This is normally approached by statistical techniques using a hypothesis-driven method [6]. Measured response is averaged over many repeated trials, also using hypotheses about the statistical distribution of response and disturbances, and correlation with the stimulus measured in order to recognize the activated areas. The main drawback of such methods is the necessity of a large number of repeated scans to enhance the signal to noise ratio and the sensitivity of the processing with respect to the statistical hypotheses applied. Moreover, only signals which belong to the specific experimental paradigm can be detected. Since unexpected phenomena, or simply delayed time-courses, are not included in the experimental hypotheses, the resulting analysis can reveal only expected activity. This is considered as a strong limitation in all experiments where stimuli cannot be characterized with respect of time, as spontaneous pathological activities or learning processes.

Data-driven methods may solve such problems more efficiently. Principal Component Analysis (PCA), Cluster Analysis, and Self-Organizing Maps have been applied, obtaining up to four-fold enhancement of signal to noise ratio, and reduced computation time. However, results are not easy interpreted and rather sensitive to some necessary choices, limiting the advantages obtained by a reduction in hypotheses. Independent Component Analysis (ICA) has been applied to BOLD-fMRI data with the aim of separating stimulated activity without making hypotheses on its temporal and/or spatial structure [7,8]. In this way, it was proved that the signal of interest is separated better than in using other methods, and that the lack of hypotheses permits other informational signals to be separated too, such as those due to heart rhythm or movement effects, opening the way to recognition of unexpected brain activations. ICA requires the definition of the expected number of independent components. If the number of independent components is lower than the actual dimensionality, after the independent components retrieval the proposed algorithm spans the subspace containing Gaussian residuals [12].

Based on these results, we conjectured that ICA is a promising method for real-time fMRI processing. In this work, we successfully applied ICA to small sets of data (i.e. using short time sequences) and compatible activities were found. Short time analysis showed an excellent ability of ICA in revealing brain activity. This may represent a crucial point for a potential extension of this technique to event-related fMRI where hemodynamic signals are not reinforced by iterated presentation of the stimulus. Moreover, computation might be realized in real time by means of dedicated and quite simple hardware. In this way, results are available during or just after the scan, diagnosis can be done earlier than usual, and the protocol may be adjusted in case the results are unsatisfactory.

2 Materials, Methods, and Experiments

2.1 Independent Component Analysis

Independent Component Analysis (ICA) is a statistical methodology developed for estimating a set of independent linearly mixed sources, which we assume the set of signals under observation is composed of. ICA is usually applied to blind source separation [9] and feature extraction [10]. A theoretical foundation of ICA can be found in [11]. The ability of ICA to extract statistically independent components by a linear mixture of signals is based on the minimization of negentropy evaluated on the observed components. An efficient neural algorithm for ICA evaluation has been proposed in [12] (Fixed Point for One Unit Algorithm). This algorithm can be described by the iterative formula:

$$\begin{cases} \mathbf{w}^+_{j+1} = E\left\{\mathbf{x} \cdot g\left(\mathbf{w}^T_j \mathbf{x}\right)\right\} - E\left\{g'\left(\mathbf{w}^T_j \mathbf{x}\right)\right\} \mathbf{w}_j \\ \mathbf{w}_{j+1} = \dfrac{\mathbf{w}^+_{j+1}}{\left|\mathbf{w}^+_{j+1}\right|} \end{cases} \qquad (1)$$

where $G(y) = \dfrac{y^4}{4}$ is an efficient choice of the contrast function (kurtosis function), $g(\bullet)$ is the derivative of $G(\bullet)$ and $g'(y) = \dfrac{dg}{dy}$. A pre-whitening operation is required in order to fulfill the algorithm hypotheses (normalized weights) and to reduce the number of freedom degrees of the ICA parameters [12]. This can be accomplished by applying a PCA transformation on the fMRI raw data. The convergence of fixed-point algorithm has been demonstrated to be global for kurtosis function. For this reason this function was used in all experiments presented in this paper.

2.2 Experimental Setup

Time series of fMRI data were acquired in one healthy individual (male, 27 yr). A Philips Vision Gyroscan MR system operating at 1.5T and equipped for echo-planar imaging was employed for acquiring anatomical and functional MR images. A circular polarized volume head coil was used for radio frequency transmission and reception. Head movement was minimized by mild restraint and cushioning. Functional T2* weighted images (25 axial slices, thickness=4mm, TR=3000ms, TE=50ms, FA=90°, FOV=240cm, 64×64 matrix, voxel dimension = 3.75mm× 3.75mm×4mm) were acquired from the participant. One data acquisition run consisted of a series of 150 such BOLD sensitive images [13]. The 6 initial BOLD images were discarded from further consideration to remove any possible influence of magnet settlement.

During acquisition, the participant executed a simple motor task consisting of self-paced, sequential finger-to-thumb opposition movements with amplitude and frequency as greater as possible.

Every motor task was 15'' long and was followed by a 15'' resting period. 14 periods of hand movement and 15 periods of rest were alternated in a block-designed paradigm, for a total time of about 7' 30''. Starting and ending of stimuli were ruled by acoustic signals transmitted to the subject through the scanner earphones.

In order to compare results given by application of ICA algorithm, we performed a preliminary analysis by processing acquired data using a hypothesis-driven method (SPM99, http://www.fil.ion.ucl.ac.uk/spm). Data were processed by performing movement correction, normalization, smoothing via Gaussian kernel and finally the application of the general linear model [14]. The results obtained by SPM (statistical threshold $p<0.05$, cluster extent $\chi_E=500$) showed suitable areas of activity corresponding to the performed motor task (controlateral and ipsilateral sensorimotor cortex, ipsilateral cerebellar cortex), as shown in Figure 1.

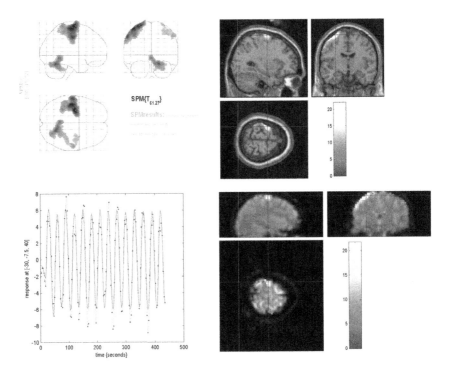

Fig. 1. SPM99 analysis result. Top-left: measured brain activity projected on a transparent model of the brain. Bottom-left: fitted model extracted by correlated voxels (red) and time evolution of maximum activation point (blue). Top-right: projection of the maximum activity on a normalized anatomic image MRI-T1 (Tailarach space). Bottom-right: projection of the maximum activity on the non-normalized image of scanned brain ($p<0.05$).

We applied a fixed-point ICA algorithm to the acquired data set. No preprocessing operation was performed on data as we expect that ICA approach is robust to parameters variation and noise influence. The only requirements we have to satisfy are related to zero mean of signals and the whitening operation with unitary autocorrelation. It is to be noted that the support of data is four-dimensional. If we order voxels spatially into a one-dimensional array, we can arrange them into a two-dimensional array that has one spatial and one temporal dimension. This array can be considered either as a set of temporal signals describing evolution at each spatial position, or a set of signals defined on space (images), taken at different times. Therefore, it is possible to perform a temporal ICA that yields ICs that have a temporal support, or a spatial ICA that yields images as result.

We tried both options to evaluate pros and cons of each. In the first case, the maximum number of ICs that can be extracted is equal to the number of measured voxels, while in the latter it is equal to number of measured time sample. In order to simplify calculation, and without loss of generality, we processed a subset of the data acquired consisting of 676 voxels taken as a connected 26×26 area of a single slice, which was known in advance to contain the maximum activation for the task considered. Using the described protocol, 144 samples in time were available. Moreover, since a volume is sampled every 3 sec. we don't expect to reveal all the physiological contributions (as heart beat or breathing) whose characteristic frequency is greater than the sampling frequency.

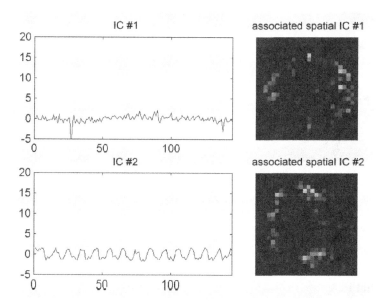

Fig. 2. Left: time course of two temporal independent components (*x*-axis: order of temporal dynamic, *y*-axis: signal amplitude). In IC #2 activation in the motor cortex is visible (other ICs behave qualitatively like IC#1). Right: associated spatial components; since ICA spatial evaluation is invariant by a generic scale factor, spatial components are represented as normalized and in absolute value format.

2.3 Temporal ICA

We started out by studying temporal ICA (tICA). When the maximum number of ICs are extracted (144), they vanish almost everywhere, except for a single narrow spike. In fact such behavior is known from literature [10]. This means that the representation obtained, even if accurate, is not significant for our purposes. Therefore, we attempted a reduction of dimensionality of the data by projecting them on their first n principal components, for variable n, and from those n PCs we extracted n ICs. We observed that when n is small, the extracted components show a significant evolution in time, and that one of them is strongly correlated with the time course of the stimulus. This correlation achieves a maximum of 0.57 when 8 components are extracted. We can check which voxels are actually active on this component by examining the unmixing matrix. In this way, it appears that such activation is in fact localized in the pertinent area of motor cortex, while activation of the other ICs is not (Figure 2).

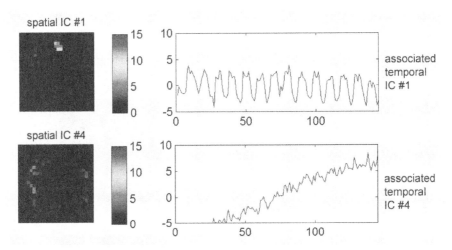

Fig. 3. Left: spatial independent components evaluated after a dimension reduction by means of PCA. Right: associated temporal components. The first component is the most correlated with the *a priori* model (box-car). Correlation factor: 0.619396.

2.4 Spatial ICA

We can apply a dual procedure to extract spatial ICs from the same data (sICA). This approach seems to be more promising with respect to the classical temporal case. Actually, magnetic resonance scanners are structurally optimized for acquiring high-quality well-defined images in comparison with a relatively low temporal sampling frequency. This characteristic is motivated by the natural application of MR to clinical imaging and the nature itself of BOLD-fMRI signals. These considerations reveal a potential efficiency improvement of ICA approach to spatial signals with respect to temporal case. Again, we extracted the maximum number of ICs. From the unmixing matrix we computed the temporal activation related to each of them and evaluated correlation with the time course of the stimulus. In this case, even without reduction of data dimensionality, we find several components that are quite correlated with the signal.

Localization of activity is again in the expected area, but the response is spread over several ICs, so that it would have been not so evident unless we knew in advance what to expect. For this reason, we tried reduction of dimensionality in this case as well. Again, when 8 ICs are extracted, one of them is strongly correlated with the stimulus (up to 0.62), and appears in the expected area, which is in this case clearly covered (Figure 3). Even if in this case dimensionality reduction does not make such a significant change in results as when temporal ICA is used, it is to be noted that there is in any case a large reduction in computation, which allows for substantial speed-up.

2.5 Real-Time Processing of fMRI Data

Hypothesis-driven methods, currently widely used in fMRI processing, are based on statistical analysis. This involves the necessity of acquiring a large amount of data before any result can be computed in order to increase the statistical population and improve, in terms of noise reduction and results reliability, the application of the general linear model. ICA-based methods, instead, seem to be a promising technique when dealing with reduced data sets. This characteristic can be considered as a direct consequence of the original independence between the components, which is a dominant feature even in small data sets. Besides, in the case of fMRI even a single image (time sample) contains a large amount of data, because sampling in space is quite dense. For these reasons, we attempted application of spatial ICA on shortened time series, using dimensionality reduction by projecting data on their first 8 PCs. We applied sICA on fMRI signals limited to some reduced time lengths. We started the first evaluation with a 30 s time length acquisition, which is the repetition time of the stimulus, i.e. the period that contains a single active and a single inactive phase. Then we increased the time length by 30 s every further evaluation. Results of correlation of ICs with the stimulus (computed as in the previous section) at selected observation lengths (Figure 4) are shown in Table 1.

Table 1. Correlation values between the eight extracted spatial independent components and the reference model (box-car). In each row, correlation at different acquisition times is shown.

	1	2	3	4	5	6	7	8
30"	0.7504	0.0000	0.2803	0.4355	0.2512	0.3246	0.3278	0.2646
120"	0.7456	0.6163	0.0000	0.0966	0.0000	0.4681	0.3054	0.3703
210"	0.6892	0.0292	0.5431	0.4213	0.6341	0.4380	0.2453	0.5076

The presented results open up the possibility of computing results of fMRI scans in real time, i.e. while it is being done. In this way, it would be possible for the operator or physician to have an immediate feeling of the content of the scan being performed, to adjust, if needed, the measurement and /or stimulation protocol, and to seek deeper insight when unexpected measured activation are observed. Of course, in order to perform a real-time fMRI data processing, the advantage given by the reduced time-windowed data set must be supported by a suitable processing resource. In fact, even if the computation required is substantially reduced with respect to statistical methods, still significant resources are needed, especially if we require that the result be available within few seconds.

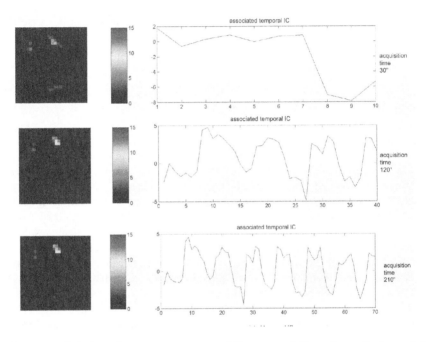

Fig. 4. Extracted independent components at different acquisition times. Left: spatial independent components. Right: associated temporal components. The first resul shown is based on just 10 temporal samples. Activity in controlateral sensorymotor cortex is well defined, in accordance with SPM99.

3 Conclusion and Discussion

Application of Independent Component Analysis to fMRI spatiotemporal data shows a great reliability in extracting hemodynamic components and identifying brain activity. The independence from strong preliminary hypotheses makes this method a fundamental starting point for all those experiments whose paradigms cannot be well-defined in terms of temporal events. It has been shown that extension of ICA to spatial data improves the ability to separate interesting components and, mainly, permits an efficient approach for real-time evaluation. Moreover, the associated temporal evolution described by the ICA linear coefficients allows a satisfactory representation of hemodynamic time course. These results support future applications of ICA to event-related fMRI where hemodynamic components are not strengthened by iterated stimuli. Furthermore, experimental paradigms devoted to identification of cognitive states such as in visual or auditory recognition (like musical themes or spoken language) may be approached by using this technique. A crucial point in ICA approach is represented by necessity to select the suitable components describing the paradigm-related signals. In our experiments, after a preliminary dimension reduction operated by PCA, the representative components have been chosen in such a way that the correlation with the box-car paradigm was as large as possible. This procedure does not satisfy the general independence from experimental hypotheses which is the main characteristic of ICA approach. Since the ICA operator is invariant upon scaling of signal amplitude, the only useful discriminating feature is represented by the informative content of signals. Anyway fMRI signals related to brain activity can be considered as a suitable superposition of hemodynamic impulse response functions, usually modeled by a combination of Gamma functions [15]. This hypothesis may be taken into account in order to estimate a representative statistical distribution, which the extracted components should be related to.

References

1. Rosen, B.R., Buckner, R.L., Dale, A.M.: Event-related functional MRI: Past, present, and future". Proc. of Natl. Acad. Sci. USA **95** (1998) 773-780
2. Arthurs, O.J., Boniface, S.: How well do we understand the neural origins of the fMRI BOLD signal?. Trends in Neurosciences **25** (2002) 27-31
3. Kwong, K., Belliveau, J.W., Chesler, D.A., Goldberg, I.E., Weisskoff, R.M., Poncelet, B.P., Kennedy, D.N., Hoppel, B.E., Cohen, M.S., Turner, T., Cheng, H.M., Brady, T.J., Rosen, B.R.: Dynamic magnetic resonance imaging of human brain activity during primary sensory stimulation. Proc. Natl. Acad. Sci. USA **89** (1992) 5675–5679
4. Iannetti, G.D., Di Bonaventura, C., Pantano, P., Giallonardo, A..T., Romanelli, P.L., Bozzao, L., Manfredi, M., Ricci, G.B.: fMRI/EEG in paroxysmal activity elicited by elimination of central vision and fixation. Neurology **58** (2002) 976-979
5. Pantano, P., Iannetti, G.D., Caramia, F., Mainero, C., Di Legge, S., Bozzao, L., Pozzilli, C., Lenzi, G.L.. Cortical motor reorganization after a single clinical attack of multiple sclerosis. Brain (2002), *in press*
6. Friston, K.J., Jezzard, P., Turner, R.: Analysis of Functional MRI Time-Series. Human Brain Mapping (1994) **1** 153-171
7. McKeown, M.J., Makeig, S., Brown, G.G., Jung, T.-P., Kindermann, S.S., Bell, A.J., Sejnowski, T.J.: Analysis of fMRI Data by Blind Separation into Independent Spatial Components. Human Brain Mapping **6** (1998), 160-188
8. Dodel, S., Herrmann, J.M., Geisel, T.: Localization of Brain Activity – Blind Separation of fMRI Data. Neurocomputing **32-33** (2000) 701-708
9. Jutten, C., Herault, J.: Blind separation of sources, Part I: An adaptive algorithm based on neuromimetic architecture. Signal Processing **24** (1991) 1–10
10. Hyvärinen, A., Oja, E., Hoyer, P., Hurri, J.: Image feature extraction by sparse coding and independent component analysis. Proc. Int. Conf. Pattern Recognition (ICPR'98), Brisbane, Australia, 1998, 1268–1273
11. Comon, P.: Independent component analysis—A new concept? Signal Processing **36** (1994) 287–314
12. Hyvärinen, A.: Fast and Robust Fixed-Point Algorithms for Independent Component Analysis. IEEE Trans. on Neural Networks, **10** (1999)
13. Kwong, K., Belliveau, J.W., Chesler, D.A., Goldberg, I.E., Weisskoff, R.M., Poncelet, B.P., Kennedy, D.N., Hoppel, B.E., Cohen, M.S., Turner, T., Cheng, H.M., Brady, T.J., Rosen,

B.R.: Dynamic magnetic resonance imaging of human brain activity during primary sensory stimulation. Proc. Natl. Acad. Sci. Usa **89** (1992) 5675–5679.
14. Friston, K.J, Holmes, A.P., Worsley, K.J., Poline, J.P., Frith, C.D., Frackowiak, R.S.J.: Statistical parametric maps in functional imaging: A general linear approach. Human Brain Mapping **2** (1995) 189-210.
15. Miezin, F. M., Maccotta, L., Ollinger, J.M., Petersen, S.E., Buckner, R.L.: Characterizing the Hemodynamic Response: Effects of Presentation Rate, Sampling Procedure, and the Possibility of Ordering Brain Activity Based on Relative Timing. Neuroimage **11** (2000) 735–759.

Implementation of an IT System for the Support of a Hospital Infection Surveillance System

Michael Behnke, Tim Eckmanns, Henning Rüden

Institut für Hygiene, FU-Berlin /
Zentralbereich Krankenhaushygiene und Infektionsprävention, HU Berlin
Heubnerweg 6
14059 Berlin, Germany
{michael.behnke tim.eckmanns henning.rueden}@charite.de

Abstract. At the national reference center for surveillance in Germany a project for the surveillance of nosocomial infections (Krankenhaus-Infektions-Surveillance-System – hospital infection surveillance system - KISS) was developed. Participants of this project are 475 intensive care units and surgical departments in the entire Federal Republic. The authors concentrate in the paper on the introduction of a IT system for the surveillance of nosocomial infections. The applications and software modules, which are important for the system, are described. Data are collected by an eCRF based surveillance program. The entered data are administered and processed in a central data base. The participants get periodically a statistic evaluation of their data.

Background

Nosocomial Infections (NI) are hospital aquired infections. They are the main factor for complications of hospital stay. The most important nosocomial infections are urinary tract infections, pneumonias, bacteraemias and surgical site infections. These infections count for ¾ of all NI in German hospitals [1].

NI are a huge threat for the patients. They often cause a prolongation of the hospital stay and in some cases they are responsible for the death during hospital stay. So it is not only a threat for the patients but also an economical problem.

The prolongation of the hospital stay costs about 500 Euro each day in average [2, 3]. Most NI are developed on intensive care units.

The problem of NI will increase because of the demographic development. The population will become older and age is a risk factor for NI. There is also a growing number of resistent bacteria which often lead to NI and the type of care in hospitals will become more aggressive, for example in oncology and haematology which will lead to more immunosuppression and subsequently to more NI [4].

For prevention of nosocomial infections the National Reference Center for Hospital Hygiene (Nationales Referenzzentrum für Krankenhaushygiene, NRZ) developed a surveillance system, Krankenhaus-Infektions-Surveillance-System (KISS) [5]. The aim of the surveillance system is to create a national database [6].

A. Colosimo et al. (Eds.): ISMDA 2002, LNCS 2526, pp. 177-185, 2002.
© Springer-Verlag Berlin Heidelberg 2002

Hospitals from all over Germany collect their NI in a standardized way and send the data to the NRZ.

Here we calculate the data individually for each hospital and calculate reference data for all hospitals. So each hospital can compare its data with the reference data and observe its own trend of infection rates over the time. In this way KISS is a important part of the quality management of the hospitals.

Objectives
- To develop an IT-based surveillance system which considers the suggestions of the hospitals
- The possibility to extend KISS for many more participants
- To reduce workload for NRZ
- To improve quality of data

Method

KISS consists of two components, one for intensive care units (ICU) with a stratification for different kinds of ICUs (surgical, medical, anaesthesia, pediatrics, neurosurgical) and one for surgical departments (Surgery). There are further surveillance systems, e.g. for neonatal intensive care units and bone marrow transplantation, in development.

In the ICU component the hospitals collect data of urinary tract infection, pneumonia, bacteremia and other nosocomial infections. In addition data for the denominator are collected (table 1). In the surgery component the hospitals collect data of surgical site infections of special procedures like appendectomy, colectomy, bypass operation etc. For the denominator all operations of the special kind are listed. Table 1 shows the parameters needed for the infection rate calculations.

Table 1. Overview of type of data.

Component	Denominator data	Cases
ICU	Kind of ICU Inlaying patients Number of patients Number of patients with urinary tract catheters Number of intubated patients Number of patients with central venous catheter	Kind of ICU Identifying code Age Sex Kind of infection Catheter yes/no Germs Secondary bacteremia Death
Surgical department	ASA-Score Wound contamination class Length of operation	Same as denominator and Kind of infection germs

With this data the following calculations were done:

For each participating ICU

- Monthly device-utilization rates for urinary tract catheters, tubus and central venouse catheter
- Monthly incidence density for urinary tract infection, pneumonia and bacteremia
- Pooled device-rates
- Pooled device-associated infection rates
- Figures

Reference data for all ICUs (each type of ICU):
- Number of wards participating
- Number of observation months
- Number of patients
- Number of patient days
- Overall device-utilization rates for urinary tract catheters, tubus and central venouse catheter
- Overall device-associated infection rates for urinary tract infections, pneumonia and bacteremia
- Figures

For each participating surgical department:
- Number of operations (overall and per risk group)
- Number of surgical site infection (overall and per risk group)
- Rate of surgical site infection (overall and per risk group)
- Rate of surgical site infection by kind of infection
- Standardized infection rate (SIR) with confidence interval
- Figures

Reference data for all surgical departments:
- Number of departments (overall and per risk group)
- Number of operations (overall and per risk group)
- Number of surgical site infections (overall and per risk group)
- 25%, median and 75% percentile of surgical site infection rate (overall and per risk group)
- Distribution of the SIR
- Figures

KISS started 1997 with 27 ICUs and 12 surgical departments participating in the project. Data were listed on paper case report forms (CRF) on the ICUs or the surgical wards. Every month the CRFs were sent to the NRZ. After an intensive procedure of validation data were entered in a mask of SAS. Every six months the reference data were calculated and sent to the hospitals.

More explanations of the KISS-method, e.g. the selection of the risk factors can be found in [7].

Problems with collecting of data by CRF:

- Waste of time and men-power. With the increase of the number of ICUs and surgical departments there was a rise of workload (table 2).
- Problems with the quality of data. Unreadable CRF, inconsistent data, missing data.
- Repeated input of data was necessary.

To consider the wishes of the participating hospitals we made an questionnaire which was sent to all hospitals in September 1998. Only 15% of the hospitals had access to the internet. So we decided to develop a eCRF based surveillance program (KrankenhausErfaSsungsSystem, KESS) which can be used in the hospitals offline. KESS works on all windows-versions.

Process

For reasons of data security the hospitals are pushed to feed only anonymous data. When the data are sent to the NRZ by emails or by diskettes they are compressed and encrypted. If data are sent by email the sender gets a confirmation.

In the NRZ the data are copied in a special directory structure. The data are checked for completeness (the other steps of validation are described in a separate paragraph).

Afterwards metadata of the local databases of the hospitals are fed into the central Server-DB (database) of NRZ in the DataManagementCenter (DMC), to get an overview of the sent data. The data of the hospitals are sent in a cumulative way. That means all older data are sent too. If there are changes or completions there is a check which data are changed or new and these data were fed into the central Server-DB.

After preparing the raw data for the export to SAS in KESS-Export the analysis of the individually data of the hospitals and the reference data starts. At the end result reports are generated in KESS-Doc in Adobe-PDF-Format. The result reports are placed at the hospitals disposal by web. The reference data are open for all web users on the NRZ homepage [8]. The individually data are only readable with a password which is sent to the hospitals by traditional letter.

Validation

The first step of data validation takes place during the input of the data. Obligation fields and system messages force the user to put in the data.

Further validations like elimination of double entry are semi-automatic by SQL-command.

At the end there is an expert-validation. The expert controls the data for textual failures. The corrected data are put into the central Server-DB by SQL-command.

These methods of automatic control of plausibility during the data input and the following step of validation generates data of a better quality than the data achieved by the traditional data entry via case report forms.

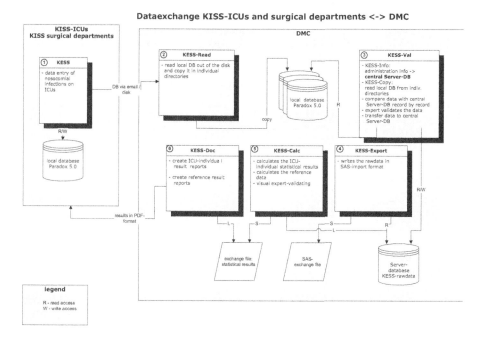

Fig. 1. The figure shows the data-flow in the KISS-IT System. The hospitals send the data to the DataManagementCenter (DMC). In the DMC the data is read and validated. After validation the data are exported to SAS a statistical software tool for further calculation (research). KESS-Calc calculates the individual and the reference results. KESS-Doc prepares the reports in Adobe-PDF-Format. Last step is the sending of the reports to the ICUs or the surgical departments.

Training and Support

All hospitals participating in KISS meet once a year for discussions about the surveillance system. We introduced KESS in the meeting in November 1999 and trained the participants in using the program. Now each year all new participants meet before starting surveillance to get a training in surveillance and KESS.

In January 2000 we installed a telephonic support. On two days a week an expert supported the users.

The most important support questions and their answers are categorized and listed under the section frequently asked questions on the homepage of the NRZ [8]. In addition there are documents and guidance for KESS and KISS itself downloadable.

Results

At present (2002) 230 ICUs and 245 surgical departments participate to KISS. A hospital usual registers several ICUs and surgical departments to KISS.

The method presented here makes an economic lead for the electronic data acquisition possible in relation to the traditional data acquisition, because by the introduction of an automated half yearly evaluation the work expended decreased substantially.

Table 2. Working time which is spend for result generating.

	Before KESS	With KESS
Mathematician	12 weeks	1 week
Secretary	2 weeks	0
Data input	12 weeks	0
Physician	12 weeks	1 week
Student	0	6 weeks
Computer scientist	0	1 week

It is possible to merge more hospitals into the KISS-project than it would have been possible due to small resources before.

Without the development of this IT-system the participation of further ICUs and surgical departments at KISS would not have been possible. Table 3 points out the development of the KISS-system since the establishment of KISS. The KESS system is in use since 2000 and since that time it is continuously extended.

Problems
A problem, which is based in the decentralized structure of the data acquisition, exists in the mixture of data of an ICUs or surgical department on different collection media. For example: an intensive care unit is sending the infection data from January to March by paper and changes the type of data entry to KESS at the beginning of March. In the DMC data are thus present, which overlap in the second half of March. A solution consists of examining the data manual. Thus an expert decides, which data are selected.

Besides it is difficult to establish program updates in all KISS participants, since here so far only the possibility of the postal report exists, but no function of an automatic update.

Clinical Effect
It is proven that the execution of the IT supported surveillance system KISS entails a significant decrease of the device-associated bloodstream infection rate [11].

Discussion

It was necessary to create a program which works on every windows platform because in the questionnaire 1998 30% of the hospitals had 3.1 or 3.11 platforms.

Table 3. Development of KISS and KESS. Numbers of ICUs and surgical departments in the years 1997 to 2003 (perspective) and information about data-collection and data-analysis in these years. KESS-Validate, KESS-Calc and KESS-Doc are explained in the text. RDE^2, DataMining and knowledge discovery will be established in future.

Time	1997	1998	1999	2000	2001	2002	perspective 2003
ICUs	23	71	127	196	212	230	250
Surgical departments	10	41	95	152	217	245	270
Datacollection	CRF[1]	CRF[1]	CRF[1]	KESS	KESS	KESS	KESS / RDE[2]
Validation	SAS[3] Expert	SAS[3] Expert	SAS[3] Expert	KESS-Validate/ SAS[3]/ Expert	KESS-Valid./ SAS[3] Expert	KESS-Valid./ SAS[3]/ Expert	KESS-Validate / RDE[2]-Val / Expert / DataMining
Routine dataanalysis	SAS[3]	SAS[3]	SAS[3]	SAS[3]	KESS-Calc	KESS-Doc	KESS-Calc / KESS-Doc / RDE /
Specialiced dataanalysis research	SAS[3]	SAS[3]	SAS[3]	SAS[3] SPSS[3]	SAS[3] SPSS[3]	SAS[3] SPSS[3]/ STATA[3]	SAS[3] / SPSS[3] / STATA[3] / DataMining / Knowledge-Discovery
Reports	Word	Word	Word	MS-Access-Reports	MS-Access-Reports	MS-Access-Reports	Reports PDF / HTML /
DBMS	SAS[3]	SAS[3]	SAS[3]	SQL-Server	SQL-Server	SQL-Server	SQL-Server

[1] Case report form
[2] Remote data entry
[3] Software for statistical data-analysis

So we had to provide a 16-Bit application. Because of memory and function delimitations of 16-Bit applications in relation to current 32-Bit applications the development became more complex.

However KESS is an Windows application, in order to give the users an actual user interface.

In the future methods are developed to minimize the temporal expenditure, which results from the manual data input. In the hospitals, in which hospital information systems and operating management systems are installed, data like e.g. the operating lists flows via an import function automatically into the data collection program. However by KISS at present the coding of the operations is expected by special indicator surgery abbreviation. So there is the problem, that by the IT departments of the participants a conversion of its standardized operation procedure code (OPS) to the special indicator surgery abbreviation must be programmed. In the future in the KISS-system OPS codes are used. For this a concept is to be developed, how to integrate the OPS codes in the KISS-system.

Altogether the satisfaction of the participants rose by the introduction of the IT-System.

Because of the usage of KESS the users receive also a tool for the hospital internal documentation of infections. They have the possibility of the subsequent treatment in other programs. The participants receive responding results for presentations of their infection rates.

The introduction of a new infection law requires the documentation of nosocomial infections in Germany. The legal documentation obligation is fulfilled by the use of KESS and the participation in KISS.

Due to the success of KISS in Germany KESS was established as quasi-standard device for the collection of NIs. A standardized import interface is compiled, so that other vendors' systems can pass their infection data on to KESS. Thus the standardisation efforts in the NRZ are developed further in the future.

In the SCENIC study it was in principle proven that clinical Surveillance reduces the NI rate [9]. SCENIC is a forerunner of the NNIS project [10] and KISS contains the substantial elements of NNIS [5]. The significant decrease of the device-associated bloodstream infection rate in KISS can be partly contributed to development in the IT sector, as there are data of higher quality and there are more possibilities for the participants to operate with their own data.

It was stated by the telephone contact with the users and further inquiries that more and more hospitals are connected to the internet. So in the future we plan a surveillance system with online remote data entry technology.

References

1. Rüden, H., et al., *Nosocomial and community-acquired infections in Germany. Summary of the results of the First National Prevalence Study (NIDEP)*. Infection, 1997. 25(4): p. 199-202.
2. Moris de la Tassa, J., et al., *[Study of costs associated with catheter-related bacteremia]*. Rev Clin Esp, 1998. 198(10): p. 641-6.
3. Merle, V., et al., *Assessment of prolonged hospital stay attributable to surgical site infections using appropriateness evaluation protocol*. Am J Infect Control, 2000. 28(2): p. 109-15.
4. Barza, M. and K. Travers, *Excess infections due to antimicrobial resistance: the "Attributable Fraction"*. Clin Infect Dis, 2002. 34(Suppl 3): p. S126-30.

5. Geffers, C., et al., *Establishment of a national database for ICU-associated infections. First results from the "Krankenhaus-Infections-Surveillance-System" (KISS).* Anaesthesist, 2000. 49(8): p. 732-7.

6. Gastmeier, P., et al., *How to survey nosocomial infections.* Infect Control Hosp Epidemiol, 2000. 21(6): p. 366-70.

7. Schulze, C., et al., *Handbuch für die Surveillance von nosokomialen Infektionen nach den Methoden des Krankenhaus-Infektions-Surveillance-Systems KISS.* 2002.

8. NRZ, *NRZ für Krankenhaushygiene, www.nrz-hygiene.de.* 2000.

9. Haley, R.W., et al., *The efficacy of infection surveillance and control programs in preventing nosocomial infections in US hospitals.* Am J Epidemiol, 1985. 121(2): p. 182-205.

10. Emori, T.G., et al., *National nosocomial infections surveillance system (NNIS): description of surveillance methods.* Am J Infect Control, 1991. 19(1): p. 19-35.

11. Zuschneid, I., et al., *Reducing central line associated primary bloodstream infections in ICUs is possible: Data from the German Nosocomial Infection Surveillance System (KISS).* Infect Control Hosp Epidemiol. In press.

An Artificial Neural Network for 3D Localization of Brainstem Functional Lesions

M. Capozza[1], G.D. Iannetti[1], J.J. Marx[2], G. Cruccu[1], N. Accornero[1]

1. Department of Neurosciences, University of Rome "La Sapienza", Italy
neri.accornero@uniroma1.it
2. University of Mainz, Germany

Abstract. The human brainstem is a highly complex structure where even small lesions can give rise to a variety of symptoms and signs. Localizing the area of dysfunction within the brainstem is often a difficult task.

To make localization easier, we have developed a neural net system, which uses 72 clinical and neurophysiological data inputs and displays it (using 5268 voxels) on a three-dimensional model of the human brainstem. The net was trained by means of a back-propagation algorithm, over a pool of 580 example-cases. Assessed on 200 test-cases, the net correctly localized 83.6% of the target voxels; furthermore the net correctly localized the lesion in 31/37 patients. Because our computer-assisted method provides a reliable and quantitative localization of brainstem areas of dysfunction and can be used as a 3D interactive functional atlas, we expect that it will prove useful as a diagnostic tool for assessing focal brainstem lesions.

1 Introduction

The human brainstem is a small structure that performs hundreds of functions. Here, in closely arranged groups lie the nuclei and rootlets of the cranial nerves, and the long pathways interconnecting the brain, cerebellum, and spinal cord. Focal lesions in the brainstem can give rise to an array of symptoms and signs. In clinical practice, localizing a brainstem lesion is often a hard task even for an expert neurologist. Although magnetic resonance imaging (MRI) is helpful, areas of abnormal MRI signal do not necessarily imply tissue damage or dysfunction. Conversely, areas of actual dysfunction may escape MRI detection. The functional correlation of MRI findings is notably poor in inflammatory diseases of the brainstem (ORMEROD *et al.*, 1986; CAPRA *et al.*, 1989; TURANO *et al.*, 1991). Neurophysiological investigations (evoked potentials and trigeminal reflexes) add important topodiagnostic information not obtainable by clinical examination alone (HOPF, 1994; KIMURA *et al.*, 1994; ONGERBOER DE VISSER and CRUCCU, 1993). But integrating the information from the various neurophysiological tests requires expert neurophysiologists with a specialized knowledge of the brainstem (CRUCCU and DEUSCHL 2000).

A. Colosimo et al. (Eds.): ISMDA 2002, LNCS 2526, pp. 186-197, 2002.

Localizing the site of brainstem dysfunction is therefore a complex task that encompasses clinical symptoms, neurophysiological responses and the possible involvement of brainstem structures.

Our aim was to solve the clinical problem of integrating all this information to help localizing focal brainstem lesions. To do so, we developed a computer-aided tool using a three dimensional (3D) model of the brainstem and a neural net. We chose a neural net because connectionist systems have proved valuable in performing arbitrary mapping between highly complex input/output spaces, while exhibiting other desirable properties such as inductive generalization and gentle degradation (FELDMAN and BALLARD, 1982; RUMELHART *et al.*, 1986; GROSSBERG, 1988; KOHONEN, 1990; SIMPSON, 1990; MILLER *et al.*, 1992; BISHOP, 1995)..

2 System Architecture

Using data from topometric and stereotactic atlases (SHALTENBRAND AND WAHEM, 1977; PAXINOS and HUANG, 1995; KRETSCHMANN and WEINRICH, 1998), we developed an idealized 3D model of the brainstem subdivided into 5268 volume elements ("voxels") ranging from 2 x 2 x 2 mm to 2 x 2 x 4 mm (Fig. 1).

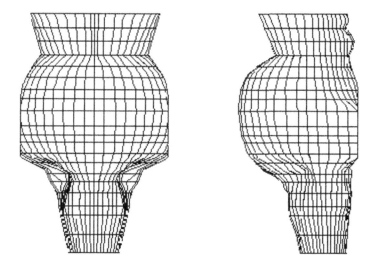

Fig. 1. Framework of the brainstem model; front view (left) and lateral view (right) (modified from Capozza et al. 2000).

Input to the neural net comprised 72 clinical and neurophysiological data items (see below and Table 1), 36 for the left side of the body and 36 for the right side, each having one of 4 possible binary values: 00 = not available; 01 = normal; 10 = abnormal; and 11 = uncertain. These values were fed into the input layer of the neural net program, which computed and output 5268 floating-point values in the range 0-1 for each of the 5268 voxels. Value 1 stood for a voxel certainly affected by the lesion, value 0 for a voxel certainly unaffected, with fractional values for intermediate probabilities (local probability of lesion, LPL) that the given voxel was affected.

Each voxel was color-coded according to its LPL and displayed at its proper location in the brainstem model, creating a 3D color map of the whole functional lesion in the brainstem (Fig. 2). This model could be freely rotated and enlarged or reduced ("zoomed") to examine the lesion from any desired angle and apparent distance. From the 3D model, 2D slices could be extracted along any of the three main section planes, and further elaborated graphically to smooth the boundaries (Fig. 3). For pictorial purposes the results can also be exported to a Computer Assisted Design and/or rendering program, such as Autocad® or 3D Studio® to be converted into a solid, smooth 3D image.

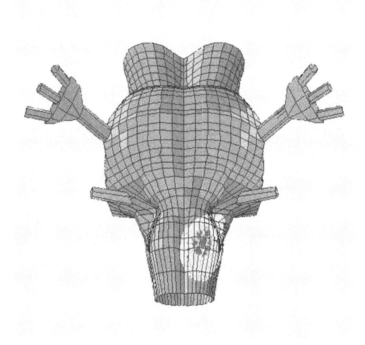

Fig. 2. 3D reconstruction of the functional lesion in a patient with a lateral medullary infarction (Wallenberg's syndrome) (modified from Capozza et al. 2000).

This software system can be run on any computer with a 24-bit color display having at least 800X600 pixel resolution, under a 32-bit Windows® operating system (Windows95®, Windows98®, WindowsNT®). The network size is about 4 Mb but 16 Mb Random Access Memory is desirable to ensure fast and smooth graphics.

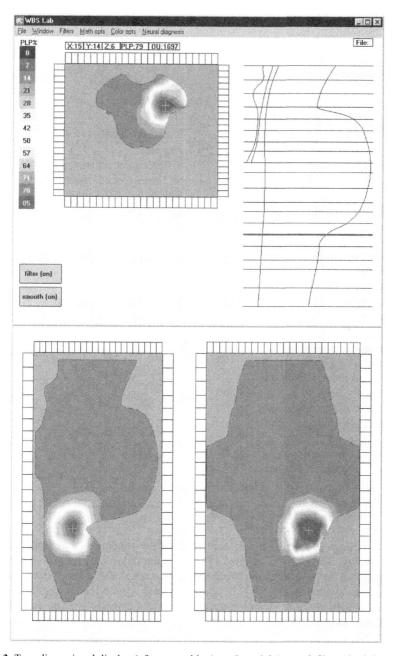

Fig. 3. Two-dimensional display (after smoothing) on the axial (upper left), sagittal (lower left), and coronal (lower right) planes, of the functional lesion shown in Figure 2. The red line on the sagittal frame (upper right) indicates the level of the axial section. The color scale represents the local probability of lesion (LPL), increasing from blue to red. The cursor in the middle of the red areas indicates the maximum LPL (79%) (modified from Capozza et al. 2000).

3 Functional Input Data

Of the 36 input data, 23 were standard clinical signs and symptoms of brainstem dysfunction (Table 1).

Table 1. Items of functional input.

Clinical examination	Neurophysiological tests
Oculomotor nerve palsy	Jaw jerk
Trochlear nerve palsy	SP1 masseter inhibitory reflex
Abducens nerve palsy	SP2 masseter inhibitory reflex
Internuclear ophthalmoplegia	SP1-SP2 crossed abnormality
Trigeminal hypesthesia	R1 blink reflex
Trigeminal pain	R2 blink reflex (afferent abnormality)
Trigeminal neuralgia	R2 blink reflex (efferent abnormality)
Facial nerve palsy	R2 blink reflex (crossed abnormality)
Hearing disturbances	BAEP* III wave
Dizziness	BAEP* V wave
Lateral propulsion	Motor evoked potentials
Nystagmus	Somatosensory evoked potentials
Rotatory nystagmus	Laser evoked potentials
Nystagmoid movements	
Dysphagia dysphonia dysarthria	
Pharyngeal reflex suppression (unilateral)	
Vocal cord palsy (unilateral)	
Accessory nerve palsy	
Hypoglossal nerve palsy	
Pyramidal syndrome	
Lemniscal sensory disturbance	
Spinothalamic sensory disturbance	
Ataxia	

*BAEP: brainstem auditory evoked potential

The 13 neurophysiological items were obtained by trigeminal reflex and evoked potential testing. The jaw jerk elicited by taps to the chin is a trigemino-trigeminal reflex mediated by a short, unilateral pontomesencephalic circuit (Cruccu and Ongerboser de Visser 1999 HOPF). The masseter inhibitory reflex elicited by perioral electrical stimulations is a trigemino-trigeminal reflex consisting of an early (SP1) and late component (SP2). SP1 is mediated by a short, bilateral, pontine circuit. SP2 is mediated by a long, bilateral, pontomedullary circuit. Impulses for the contralateral response cross at the level of the pontomedullary junction (Cruccu and Ongerboser de Visser 1999 ODV et al Brain). The blink reflex elicited by electrical stimulation of the supraorbital nerve is a trigemino-facial reflex consisting of an early (R1) and a late (R2) component. R1 is a mediated by a short, unilateral pontine circuit. R2 is mediated by a long, bilateral medullary (down to the caudal medulla-rostral spinal cord) circuit. Impulses cross in the mid medulla, at the level of the obex (Cruccu and

Deuschl 2000; ODV and Cruccu 1993). The brainstem auditory evoked potentials, evoked by acoustic stimuli and recorded from the scalp, consist of several far-field waves: wave III is generated in the lower pons, wave IV in the lateral lemniscus, and wave V in the lower colliculus (Deuschl and Eisen 1999). The motor evoked potentials are elicited in facial and limb muscles by transcranial magnetic stimulation of the motor cortex. The descending volleys travel along the corticobulbar and corticospinal tracts in the ventral brainstem (Deuschl and Eisen 1999). The somatosensory evoked potentials are evoked by electrical stimulation of the median or tibial nerves and recorded from the scalp. The ascending volleys travel along the dorsal columns up to the dorsal medulla, then are relayed to the medial lemniscus, cross the midline and ascend in the brainstem tegmentum up to the thalamus (Deuschl and Eisen 1999). The laser evoked potentials are evoked by laser stimulation of the hairy skin. The ascending volleys travel in the spinothalamic tract through the whole caudal-rostral brainstem tegmentum, without crossing the midline (Arendt-Nielsen 1994; Bromm and Treede 1991).

4 Preparation of the Example-Cases and Test-Cases

To train the net, we prepared 780 example-cases, representative of the main possible combinations of symptoms and neurophysiological findings, and of the most typical brainstem lesions. All cases had one focal lesion alone.

We used a two-step process. First, we collected images of focal brainstem lesions from the existing literature and transposed them on our brainstem model. For each case we assigned to each voxel a local probability of lesion (LPL), on a three-value scale: 0 = unaffected; 0.5 = uncertain; and 1 = affected. These voxels were the target array of the neural net for that case. The input data of each case were also fed with the available clinical-neurophysiological information. Second, we submitted the cases (with both the probabilities of lesion and clinical-neurophysiological information) to three experts in brainstem anatomy and brainstem neurophysiology, who were asked to judge whether the lesion and the functional data of each case were indeed compatible. The cases approved by the experts were finally accepted for the net training.

Of the 780 example-cases, a total 200 cases were chosen randomly and transferred from the training set to the test set [ref], the remaining 580 example-cases constituted the training set.

5 Network Topology and Training

We chose a multi-layered, feed-forward, fully-connected neural network with two hidden layers, trained by back-propagation (RUMELHART et al., 1986).

The net had 148 input units (because the 74 input data were binary coded), 50 units in the first hidden layer, 150 units in the second hidden layer, and 2634 units in the output layer. By exploiting the functional right-left symmetry of the brainstem (HARNAD et al., 1977) and a two-step process, we were able to reduce the output units to one half the 5268 voxels in the model: in a first step, the net, fed with all the right and left input data, computed the output values for the left-sided voxels: in a second step the net was fed with right-left inverted input data, and the output values, right-left inverted, were assigned to the right-sided voxels.

The net used a linear transfer function from the input layer to the first hidden layer and a sigmoid function for the other layers.

The net was trained until every voxel's LPL came within 0.25 of the target value.

To train the net we used the commercial program Qnet® 2.1, which allowed automatic adjustment of the learning rate. On a Pentium II 350 MHz computer, working night and day, training took about one month.

6 Results

When training stopped the root mean square of the output error had stabilized at a level lower than 0.002. The correlation between the targets and outputs in the training set reached 0.999 (R correlation coefficient).

We also cross-validated the net with the set of 200 "unknown" test cases that had been randomly chosen and excluded from the training set (see above). The LPL error "e" for each single voxel was computed as: e = output value minus target value. False positive errors ranged from 0 to 1 and false negative errors ranged from 0 to -1. Error frequencies were grouped into classes 0.25 wide (Table 2). More than 80% of voxels (83.6%) showed an absolute error lower than 0.25.

Table 2. Distribution of error frequencies

Error (e)	Number of voxels	% of voxels
$-1 < e \leq -0.75$	0	0
$-0.75 < e \leq -0.50$	15593	1.48
$-0.50 < e \leq -0.25$	93665	8.89
$-0.25 < e < 0$	413117	39.21
$0 \leq e < 0.25$	467482	44.37
$0.25 \leq e < 0.50$	55209	5.24
$0.50 \leq e < 0.75$	8534	0.81
$0.75 \leq e < 1$	0	0
Total	1053600	100

This kind of error evaluation lacks spatial information (see Discussion). To provide information on the spatial errors, we also computed, for any voxel having an output value 'V' with an absolute error higher than 0.25, its spatial distance from the nearest voxel having a target value within ± 0.25 from 'V'. Out of 173001 voxels having absolute errors equal to or higher than 0.25, 131481 (76%) showed a spatial distance of 1 voxel (neighboring voxels) and 38060 (22%) a distance of 2 voxels. This distinction suggests that apparently high errors might in reality reflect relatively small spatial displacements in the LPL (98% were located within 2 voxels).

After net validation with the set of test-cases, we tried the method in a retrospective study of 40 patients from our neurological division. We selected patients with one focal brainstem lesion and excluded patients with multiple sclerosis or tumors, who are expected to yield a poor anatomical-functional correlation. The net was fed with the available clinical and neurophysiological data of each case. The 3D functional lesion produced by our net was submitted to the opinion of an expert who compared it with the clinical notes and the available neuroimaging pictures.

The expert judged the output of the net correct in 31 cases. In six cases, only having clinical and neurophysiological signs of impairment of the motor or sensory pathways on one side (unilateral pyramidal or somatosensory syndromes), the net assigned a uniformly low LPL to all the voxels of the involved corticospinal or somatosensory tract. In three cases the expert judged the input data insufficient

7 Discussion

While neural networks are by no means a novelty in automated diagnostic systems (SHARPE and CALEB, 1994; YANG et al., 1994; ACCORNERO and CAPOZZA, 1995; ARMONI, 1998), the diagnostic task presented is unusual because it entails topographic rather than semantic diagnosis. In conventional diagnostic systems, numerical outputs represent the likelihood that the various nosographic entities considered will be true in the observed subject. In our system, instead of an "abstract" nosographic probability, each probability had to be assigned a small, well localized spatial point in a nervous system. Quantitatively, this difference raised the number of outputs from several tens to several thousands. From a more conceptual point of view, it also required the diagnostic system to solve interesting problems about the spatial relations among the various outputs. These exigencies led us to decide against a traditional expert system and use a connectionist system.

To keep the neural net size small we applied a solution that had proved useful in an earlier study (ACCORNERO and CAPOZZA, 1995). Because, unlike the cerebral hemispheres, brainstem functions are right-left symmetric (HARNAD et al., 1977), we decided to use a net that diagnosed only one side of the brainstem, covering the entire organ by activating the net a second time after exchanging input and output data sides. The number of input units remained unchanged, because the net obviously needed to be "aware" of the clinical and neurophysiological data from both sides of the body at any single activation. This procedure halved the number of output units, thus reducing the amount of memory required. Economy was not the only reason for this arrangement. To a net considering a single side of the brainstem, each example case had a double value, because it provided two examples, one for the left and one for the right side. This resulted in virtually doubling the size of the example set.

We binary coded the 74 input data. Because the input data ranged on 4 possible categories, each input needed 2 bits and the number of input units was therefore 148. The alternative, coding each datum as a single real number, seemed unacceptable because it would have implied the use of an interval scale to encode the 4 possible values, i.e. an interval relation between nominal values. After empirical tests using a wide range of values, the number of hidden units was kept as small as possible to facilitate generalization (ANSHELEVICH et al., 1989; BAUM and HAUSSLER, 1989). The 2634 output units were obviously determined by the number of voxels required for each half of our brainstem model.

A point of importance in assessing the net's performance is that any spatial error may lead to a double LPL error. Let us assume, for example, that a given voxel had a target LPL value of 1, but the net assigned that value to a neighboring voxel, and a different value to the given voxel. This would result in a double LPL error (one in the given voxel and one in the neighboring voxel). In this example, the network software correctly computed the LPL quantitatively, but instead of assigning it to the correct voxel erroneously shifted it to a neighboring voxel. Assessing these spatial errors was difficult, because we had no way of finding out whether the net's LPL for a given voxel was actually a 'shifted' value. Nor could we identify the 'original' voxel for that value, if any. Hence, we had to verify whether any mistaken voxel (i.e. any voxel having an absolute error equal or higher than 0.25) was located within a distance of 1 or 2 voxels from another location where that value would have been acceptable (i.e. absolute error lower than 0.25). This analysis showed that most grossly mistaken voxels were spatial errors from neighboring voxels (98% when considering neighbors up to a distance of 2 voxels, i.e. 4 mm).

Unlike some other studies designed to solve a clinical problem by applying a neural net approach, in assessing the reliability of the net we could not use real patients as test-cases. Traditionally, anatomical-functional correlation studies have always relied on pathological findings. To collect a sufficient number of autopsies was beyond the scope of this study. Furthermore, the wide time interval elapsing between the functional examination and death may corrupt the findings (MASIYAMA, 1985; ONGERBOER DE VISSER et al., 1990). Although MRI is far more readily available and timely, it often provides an insufficient correlation between the areas of abnormal signal and the actual areas of dysfunction in the brainstem (BYRNE et al., 1989; CAPRA et al., 1989; CRUCCU and DEUSCHL, 1999). Indeed, the search for a way to overcome the poor ability of MRI in localizing and quantifying the *functional* lesion in some diseases prompted us to develop this project. Instead, we relied on net cross-validation with the test-cases subtracted from the training set. We also asked an expert to test *qualitatively* how the net performed on a retrospective group of patients with focal brainstem lesions secondary to diseases that are expected to provide a good anatomical/functional correlation. The net performed well. As well as yielding the correct output in most cases it failed only when it received too few data. In particular, when the patient had only dysfunction of the ascending or descending pathways in the ventral brainstem, unaccompanied by a clinical or neurophysiological abnormality indicating the cranial nerves or nuclei or the reflex pathways in the dorsal brainstem, the net could not locate the lesion rostral-caudally and assigned a low probability distributed along the pathway. Human experts have exactly the same difficulty.

In a future study we intend to compare quantitatively the correlation between the areas of abnormal signal yielded by MRI with the areas of dysfunction yielded by our neural network, in patients with ischemic infarction (expected to provide a good correlation) and in patients with multiple sclerosis (expected to provide a poor correlation).

Table 3. Items of functional input.

Clinical examination	Neurophysiological tests
Oculomotor nerve palsy	Jaw jerk
Trochlear nerve palsy	SP1 masseter inhibitory reflex
Abducens nerve palsy	SP2 masseter inhibitory reflex
Internuclear ophthalmoplegia	SP1-SP2 crossed abnormality
Trigeminal hypesthesia	R1 blink reflex
Trigeminal pain	R2 blink reflex (afferent abnormality)
Trigeminal neuralgia	R2 blink reflex (efferent abnormality)
Facial nerve palsy	R2 blink reflex (crossed abnormality)
Hearing disturbances	BAEP* III wave
Dizziness	BAEP* V wave
Lateral propulsion	Motor evoked potentials
Nystagmus	Somatosensory evoked potentials
Rotatory nystagmus	Laser evoked potentials
Nystagmoid movements	
Dysphagia dysphonia dysarthria	
Pharyngeal reflex suppression (unilateral)	
Vocal cord palsy (unilateral)	
Accessory nerve palsy	
Hypoglossal nerve palsy	
Pyramidal syndrome	
Lemniscal sensory disturbance	
Spinothalamic sensory disturbance	
Ataxia	

*BAEP: brainstem auditory evoked potential

References

ACCORNERO, N., and CAPOZZA, M. (1995): 'OPTONET: neural network for visual field diagnosis', *Med. Biol. Eng. Comput.*, **33**, pp. 223-226

ANSHELEVICH, V.V., AMIRIKIAN, B.R., LUKASHIN, A.V., and FRANK-KAMENETSKII, M.D. (1989): 'On the ability of neural networks to perform generalization by induction', *Biol. Cybern.*, **61**, pp. 125-128

ARENDT-NIELSEN, L. (1994): 'Characteristics, detection and modulation of laser-evoked vertex potentials', *Acta Anaesthesiol. Scand.*, **38**, pp. 1-36

ARMONI, A. (1998): 'Use of neural networks in medical diagnosis', *MD Comput.*, **15** (2), pp. 100-104

BAUM, E. B. and D. HAUSSLER (1989): 'What size net gives valid generalization?' *Neural Comput.*, **1** (1), pp. 151-160

BISHOP, M.C. (1995): 'Neural Networks for Pattern Recognition' (Oxford University Press, New York)

BROMM, B. and TREEDE, R.D. (1991): 'Laser evoked potentials in the assessment of cutaneous pain sensitivity in normal subjects and patients. *Rev. Neurol.*, **147**, pp. 625-643

BYRNE, J.V., KENDALL, B.E., KINGSLEY, D.P., MOSELEY, I.F. (1989): 'Lesions of the brain stem: assessment by magnetic resonance imaging', *Neuroradiology*, 31 (2), pp. 129-133

CAPLAN, L., GUTMANN, L., BESSER, R., HOPF, H.C. (1993): 'Brain-Stem Localization and Function' (Springer, Heidelberg/New York)

CAPOZZA M, IANNETTI GD, MOSTARDA M, CRUCCU G; ACCORNERO N (2000). 3D mapping of brainstem functional lesions. *Med Biol Eng Comput* **38 pp.** 639-644.

CAPRA, R., MATTIOLI, F., VIGNOLO, L.A., ANTONELLI, A.R., BONFIOLI, F., CAPPIELLO, J., NICOLAI, P., PERETTI, G. and ORLANDINI, A. (1989): 'Lesion detection in MS patients with and without clinical brainstem disorders: magnetic resonance imaging and brainstem auditory evoked potentials compared', *Eur. Neurol.* **29** (6), pp. 317-322

CRUCCU, G., and DEUSCHL G. (2000): 'The clinical use of brainstem reflexes and hand-muscle reflexes', *Clin. Neurophysiol.*, **111**, pp. 371-387

CRUCCU, G., and ONGERBOER DE VISSER, B.W. (1999): 'The jaw reflexes', *Electroencephalogr. Clin. Neurophysiol.*, suppl. **52**: pp. 243-247

DEUSCHL, G., and EISEN, A. (Eds., 1999): 'Recommendations for the Practice of Clinical Neurophysiology: Guidelines of the International Federation of Clinical Neurophysiology (2nd ed)' (Elsevier, Amsterdam)

FELDMAN, J., and BALLARD, D. (1982): 'Connectionist models and their properties', *Cognitive Sci.*, **6**, pp. 205-254

GROSSBERG, S. (1988): 'Nonlinear neural networks: principles, mechanisms, and architectures', *Neural Networks*, **1**, pp. 17-61

HARNAD, S., DOTY, R.W., GOLDSTEIN, L., JAYNES, J., KRAUTHAMER, G. (1977): 'Lateralization in the nervous system' (Academic Press, New York)

HOPF, H.C. (1994): 'Topodiagnostic value of brain stem reflexes', *Muscle Nerve*, **17**, pp. 475-484

KIMURA, J., DAUBE, J., BURKE, D., HALLETT, M., CRUCCU, G.,   ONGERBOER DE VISSER, B.W., YANAGISAWA, N., SHIMAMURA, M.,   ROTHWELL, J. (1994): 'Human reflexes and late responses. Report of an IFCN committee', *Electroencephalogr. Clin. Neurophysiol.* **90**, pp. 393-403

KOHONEN, T. (1990) The self-organizing map. *P. IEEE*, **78**, pp. 1464-1480

KRETSCHMANN, H.J., and WEINRICH, W. (1998): 'Neurofunctional Systems – 3D Reconstructions with Correlated Neuroimaging' (George Thieme Verlag, Stuttgart)

MASIYAMA, S., NIIZUMA, H., SUZUKI, J. (1985): 'Pontine haemorrhage: a clinical analysis of 26 cases', *J. Neurol. Neurosurg. Psychiatry*, **48**, pp. 658-662

MILLER, A.S., BLOTT, B.H. and HAMES, T.K. (1992): 'Review of neural network applications in medical imaging and signal processing', *Med. Biol. Eng. Comput.*, **30**, pp. 449-464

ONGERBOER DE VISSER, B.W., CRUCCU, G., MANFREDI, M., KOELMAN, J.H. (1990): 'Effects of brainstem lesions on the masseter inhibitory reflex. Functional mechanisms of reflex pathway', *Brain,* **113** (3), pp. 781-792

ONGERBOER DE VISSER, B.W., and CRUCCU, G. (1993): 'Neurophysiologic examination of the trigeminal, facial, hypoglossal, and spinal accessory nerves in cranial neuropathies and brain stem disorders' *in* BROWN, W.F., and BOLTON, C.F. (Eds.): 'Clinical Electromyography (2nd ed)' (Butterworth-Heinemann, Boston) pp. 61-92

ORMEROD, I.E., ROBERTS, R.C., DU BOULAY, E.P., MCDONALD, W.I., CALLANAN, M.M., HALLIDAY, A.M., JOHNSON, G., KENDALL, B.E., LOGSDAIL, S.J. and MACMANUS, D.G. (1984): 'NMR in multiple sclerosis and cerebral vascular disease', *Lancet* **8415** (2), pp. 1334-1335

PAXINOS, G., HUANG, X.F. (1995): 'Atlas of the human brainstem' (Academic Press, San Diego)

RUMELHART, D.E., HINTON, G.E. and WILLIAMS, R.J. (1986): 'Learning internal representations by error propagation' *in* RUMELHART, D.E. and MCCLELLAND, J.L. (Eds.): 'Parallel Distributed Processing: explorations in the microstructure of cognition. Vol. 1 (Foundations)' (MIT Press, Cambridge, Massachusetts) pp. 318-362

SHALTENBRAND, G. and WAHEM, W. (1977): 'Atlas for stereotaxy of the human brain' (Thieme, Stuttgart)

SHARPE, P.K. and CALEB, P. (1994): 'Artificial neural networks within medical decision support systems', *Scand. J. Clin. Lab. Invest. Suppl.,* **219**, pp. 3-11

SIMPSON, P.K. (1990): 'Artificial Neural Systems' (Pergamon Press, New York)

TURANO, G., JONES, S.J., MILLER, D.H., DU BOULAY, G.H., KAKIGI, R., and MCDONALD, W.I. (1991): 'Correlation of SEP abnormalities with brain and cervical cord MRI in multiple sclerosis', *Brain* **114** (Pt 1B), pp. 663-81

YANG, T.F., DEVINE, B. and MACFARLANE, P.W. (1994): 'Artificial neural networks for the diagnosis of atrial fibrillation', *Med. Biol. Eng. Comput.* **32**, (6), pp. 615-619

Dependent Rendering: Visualizing Multiple Properties of an Object

Sebastian Löbbert and Steffen Märkle

Department of Computer Graphics,
Technische Universität Berlin
Berlin, Germany
`sebal@cs.tu-berlin.de, maerkle@ieee.org`

Abstract. In this paper, a framework for visualizing multiple properties of an object by dependent rendering of data sets of two different properties is presented. The main goal of this framework is to interactively explore a data set by showing a combined 3D image of both properties. The combined rendering reveals dependencies between these properties and allows for both a good overview and a precise location of features. The framework is not constrained to any special domain of data sets and allows for a vast variety of combinations of properties. It is well suited for functional imaging in medicine and biology where one property is given by the anatomy of the object and another by the functional information. One of the properties of the object is defined as a spatial reference for the other – the dependent – property. Both properties are rendered, with the dependent property in dependence of the reference property. For the reference property, volume rendering is used, for the dependent property a variety of rendering techniques can be applied. The resulting combined rendering image is a projection of both properties at the same time.

1 Introduction

During the past 20 years, tomographic imaging methods have become a standard technique for medical diagnostics. *Magnetic Resonance Imaging* (MRI) and *Computed Tomography* (CT) are standard means to measure anatomical information. More recently, in order to measure functional information (e.g. brain activity), techniques like *functional MRI* (fMRI) and *Positron Emission Tomography* (PET), have been introduced. Another emerging technique for gathering functional information on the brain is *MagnetoEncephaloGraphy* (MEG), which measures magnetic flows induced by electrical currents in the brain.

To visualize the anatomical information from MRI and CT, several powerful techniques have been developed and established, e.g. *surface* and *volume rendering*. These techniques have been adapted to additionally visualize functional information, but there still are significant weaknesses. These weaknesses are discussed in this paper and a technique to overcome some of them is presented.

The technique described in this paper can be used in other than medical imaging contexts, therefore we will use a more general notation for some terms:

A. Colosimo et al. (Eds.): ISMDA 2002, LNCS 2526, pp. 198–209, 2002.

It is supposed that some *properties* of an *object* are examined. In the medical context, the object would be a (part of the) human body and one property its anatomy (i.e. the matter distribution), other properties would be the temperature distribution, the distribution of electrical currents originating from an epileptic source, or brain activities evoked by some action performed by the patient. Throughout this paper, the term *volume* denotes a data set containing a three-dimensional array of sampled values of one property of an object.

Unfortunately, many properties (e.g. a temperature distribution) cannot be visualized meaningfully without using a second property (e.g. the anatomical information) as a spatial reference. Otherwise, it is impossible to precisely locate features in the non-anatomic property. It is therefore neccessary to visualize both properties simultaneously. However, while for visualizing a single property of an object, especially the matter distibution, the application of volume rendering is well researched, little is known about how to visualize several properties simultaneously.

Visualizing multiple properties is also called visualizing *attributed volume data* [1] or *multi-dimensional volumes* [2], where the term multi-dimensional relates to property and not to spatial dimensions. Often, also the term *multi-modal volume data set* is applied, but this is imprecise because multi-modal means that the data sets have been acquired by different measurement techniques, this does not imply that different properties have been acquired. E.g., a CT and a MRI data set of one object represent a multi-modal pair of data sets, but essentially describe the same property (the matter distribution). On the other hand, different properties of an object are usually acquired by different modalities, therefore the term multi-modal is almost always true for data sets describing multiple properties.

In this article, a framework for visualizing two or more properties of an object in a single projection image is described. The framework is based on the assumption that one property can serve as a spatial reference and the other properties must be visualized in dependence of this reference property.

The remaining part of the paper is organized as follows: First, existing methods for visualizing multiple properties of an object are shortly discussed. Then, the requirements for a framework for visualizing multiple properties of an object are defined. Thereafter, a framework developed based on these requirements is presented. The framework is then compared to the requirements and discussed. Finally, conclusions are derived.

Although all of the following can be extended to more than two properties of an object, the description in the remainder of the paper will be restricted to two properties for the sake of simplicity.

2   Existing Approaches

Tomographic imaging facilities produce stacks of image slices of the object. These slices are usually combined into a three-dimensional grid of image data samples.

Existing visualization approaches can be classified into two categories: Visually realistic and model-based techniques. A visually realistic approach tries to produce images that look like what the examiner sees when looking at or opening the object, in the medical context these images would show what a pathologist sees when dissecting the body.

Model-based approaches do not try to produce visually realistic images but provide the user with as much information as possible by visualizing certain particularities in a visually irrealistic but well-defined and therefore comprehensible manner. In contrast to visually realistic techniques, model-based approaches allow measurements inside the model, e.g. of a tumor's size.

Three common approaches will be described in the following. They all assume that there is one base property, usually the matter distribution of the object, and, quasi as an attribute of this base property, a second property.

The *image gallery* approach shows three perpendicular cutting planes through the object. Especially in medical imaging, it is very common to show images of the matter distibution on three perpendicular planes through the object. By moving the planes, the object can be explored. This approach is basically visually realistic, as the images show cutting planes through the body as the pathologist would see them when cutting the body into slices. Additional properties, as for example neural activity, are visualized by highlighting them on these planes. This is a pure 2D-approach which requires the user to mentally reconstruct the 3D-scene from the three planes. Although allowing for a precise location of features, this approach is limited in that the second property must be quite sparse.

The *surface mapping* approach, as described by e.g. [2], maps a second property on a surface extracted from the first property. These surfaces are rendered using surface rendering, which tries to yield images similar to what the pathologist would see when dissecting the body. Unfortunately, it is not possible to gain information on the distribution of the properties below the surface using such renderings. Therefore, this approach is of little diagnostic use.

Direct volume rendering is a model-based approach which mimics the physical effects of the interaction of light and matter (especially reflection and attenuation). It is assumed that the volume represents the particles the object consists of. By using realistic values for all particles in the volume, realistic images (similar to those created by surface rendering) can be created. By changing the light absorption attributes of classes of particles, parts of the object can be left out or depicted as translucent: The image can contain information on different particularities and hence is of more use to a user who is familar with the underlying model.

For the visualization of activated regions in the brain, [3] propose direct volume rendering for the matter distribution with a transfer function to highlight activated regions. To increase the spatial understanding, they expand this technique to their *magic mirrors* approach by rendering the object from several directions and placing these additional renderings into a scene around the object's main rendering. The transfer function approach and its derivatives require the second property to be sparse and of a low dynamic range.

To conclude, the existing approaches suffer from three main weaknesses: The spatial extension and dynamic range of the second property are limited. Furthermore, only little information about the spatial constitution of the second property is delivered. Third, by regarding the second property only as an attribute of the anatomy, these approaches do not intentionally support the investigation of the second property as a subject on its own.

3   Requirements

The objective of the framework described here is to visualize two properties of an object avoiding the drawbacks of existing methods. One of these properties will usually be some kind of matter distribution, this is the only property that can be visualized by realistic images. All other properties are not visible to humans and therefore cannot be visualized realistically. Hence, a model-based approach must be applied.

In particular, the following requirements were identified for the framework:

1. Localization: Features in the properties must be precisely spatially localizable.
2. Measurability: It must be possible to virtually measure the values of one property at a given location in the other property, e.g. the electric current at a given point in the brain.
3. Arbitrary properties: The framework must allow to render as many kinds of properties as possible - it may not be restricted to certain kinds of properties.
4. Data sets of different sizes and resolutions must be usable.
5. Any property can be an entire volume: One of the major drawbacks of other systems are their limitations regarding the second property: The second property often must be sparse and of a small dynamic range. The developed framework must be able to render two entire volumes.
6. Exploration: Data sets with unknown content must be explorable.
7. No need for segmentation: The framework should be suitable for unsegmented data.
8. 3D-impression: The renderings should allow for easy mental 3D-reconstruction of the scene.
9. Relations between properties: For a given feature in one property, it must be possible to easily recognize an eventually related feature in the other property.
10. Interactivity: The framework must allow for interactive usage.

The framework described in the next section will realize these requirements.

4   The Framework

Before presenting the core algorithm of the framework, it is neccessary to explain two essential principles the framework relies on.

4.1   Essential Principles

From the above requirements, two essential principles can be derived:

1. There is always one property that can serve as spatial reference for the others.
2. Each property is a volume in its own right.

Principle 1: There Is Always a Reference Property   When visualizing an arbitrary property of an object, the observer is interested in finding some kind of features. The features then must be spatially localized: The observer has to recognize where a given feature is located in the object. This is intuitively achieved when the property represents some kind of matter, e.g. when the observer is looking for tissue with certain characteristics that indicate cancer. But when studying, for example, the distribution of electrical currents in the brain of an epilepsy patient, visualizing only the current distribution is useless because the observer has no spatial reference to where in the brain the interesting currents are that he found. This is an example of a property that, when visualized alone, has no indications for the observer about spatial locations, and even if the oberserver can find interesting features in this stand-alone visualization, they are worthless without a spatial localisation of these features.

Therefore, such properties must be visualized together with another property that serves as a spatial reference.

The spatial reference usually will be given by some kind of matter representation because matter is the property that humans are most familiar with at mentally reconstructing and bringing into a spatial context. For the rare case where there is no matter distribution available, there is always one property that the observer is more familiar with than the other, and this one will serve as the reference.

In the framework, the authors will define the property that serves as spatial reference as the *reference property* and any other property as a *dependent property* because it will be visualized in dependence of the reference property, which will be described in detail in Section 4.2. Accordingly, the term *reference volume* denotes the volume of the reference property and the *dependent volume* denotes the volume of the dependent property.

The spatial dimensions of the dependent property's data set must not exceed the spatial dimension of the reference data set – otherwise there is no spatial reference for the dependent structures and it is impossible to precisely localize features in the dependent structure.

Principle 2: A Property Is an Entire Volume   To construct a general framework, it is neccessary to be able to use data sets of arbitrary size (while, of course, obeying to the above mentioned prerequisite that no data set's size is larger than the reference property's data set's size). Data sets of properties that are defined only in parts of the reference property's size can easily be adapted to this condition by treating this property as transparent at all locations where it is not defined.

Other approaches, as for example defining a transfer function for the additional properties, are too restrictive for general use.

4.2   The Algorithm

This section describes the main processing steps of the algorithm, as depicted in Figure 1. In the following discussion, it is assumed that first, the size of the

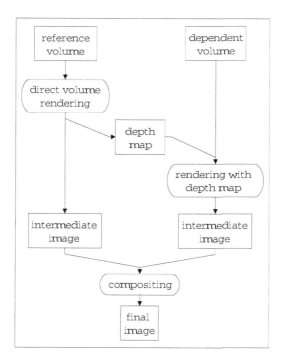

Fig. 1. The framework's main processing steps

projection image is determined from the size of the data sets. Then, three equally dimensioned data arrays are set up (see Figure 1). One for the image pixels from the reference property, one for the image pixels from the dependent property, and a third one which the authors call *depth map* and whose purpose will be described later.

In Section 4.1, it was identified as key to the understanding of many properties that they are visualized together with a spatial reference property. This must be accounted for when designing an algorithm. The key idea is to start by rendering the reference structure. Therefore, for each pixel a viewing ray is sent into the reference volume and the depth at which the viewing ray becomes opaque (i.e. the "early ray termination" point in raytracing [4]) is tracked by writing it to the depth map's entry that corresponds to this pixel.

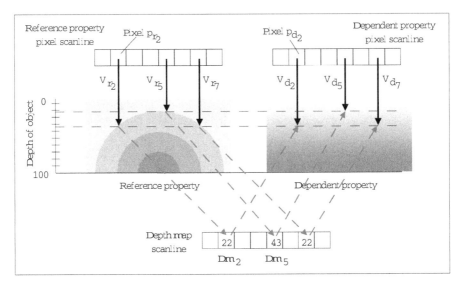

(a) Reference property classified as rather opaque

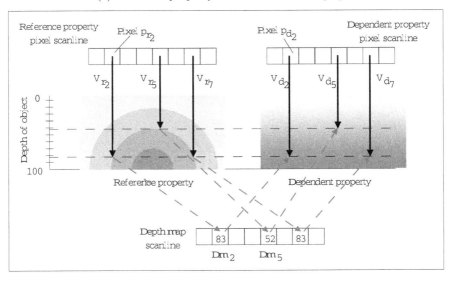

(b) Reference property classified as rather transparent

Fig. 2. Interaction of viewing rays and depth map

Then the other property is rendered, but only the parts between the viewing point and the termination depth in the reference property are taken into account, i.e. if the viewing ray for a pixel in the reference structure terminates at a depth d, the depth map entry for this pixel is set to d. In the dependent structure, this pixel's viewing ray is terminated either if it becomes fully opaque or if its depth reaches the value of its corresponding depth map entry, depending on which occurs first.

Figuratively speaking, the point where the viewing ray stops is a fully opaque wall, one cannot see what is behind this wall. In the dependent property, contributions from behind this wall would have no corresponding spatial reference from the reference structure and could therefore not be located. This is why there may be no contributions from "behind the wall".

The interaction of viewing rays, pixels and the depth map is depicted in Figures 2(a) and (b). In this simple example, a part of a slice through the volumes of two properties of an object is shown. Both volumes use the same grid spacing and coordinate system, the object has a depth of 100 units. First, viewing rays are cast into the reference volume for each pixel in the reference volume's rendering image (viewing rays V_{r_2}, V_{r_5} and V_{r_7} in the figure). The depth at which these viewing rays become opaque (for Figure 2(a) at 22, 43, and 22 units, respectively) is written to the depth map. Then, for each pixel in the dependent property's rendering image, a viewing ray is cast into the dependent volume (viewing rays V_{d_2}, V_{d_5} and V_{d_7} in the figure) and terminated when it reaches the depth given in the depth map, i.e. the depth at which the respective viewing ray in the reference volume becomes fully opaque.

In Figure 2(a), the reference property has been classified as rather opaque (the penetration depth of the viewing rays into the reference volume is quite small), whereas in Figure 2(b) the reference property has been classified as rather transparent (the penetration depth of the viewing rays into the reference volume is larger). For both examples, the dependent property has been classified such that a viewing ray transversing the whole dependent volume never becomes fully opaque. The figure shows that the penetration depth of a viewing ray in the dependent property is determined by the penetration depth of the respective viewing ray in the reference property. Thus by classifying the reference property as more or less transparent, the observer can look more or less far into the object.

The two resulting projection images can now be combined. In various tests, the authors received the best results by using intensity images with a different color for each of the properties and blending these together with an interactive mixer. This enables users to easily give the one or the other property more emphasis in the projection image.

The reference property's pixel array and the depth map must have the same size, but the dependent property's pixel array may be differently sized. For example, if the spatial resolution of the dependent volume is lower than that of the reference volume, fewer viewing rays may be sent into the dependent volume. The depth map entries then must be interpolated accordingly for each viewing ray in the dependent volume.

5 Fulfilment of Requirements

In this section, it will be investigated how well the framework fulfils the requirements defined in Section 3. Figure 3 shows two example images generated by our implementation using an MRI scan of a human head and an artificial second property consisting of a small ball of constant density located inside the brain.

Two of the requirements – any kind of properties, and a property is an entire volume – are fulfiled. They have been discussed in depth in Section 4.2.

1. Localization: The possibility to locate features of the dependent property in terms of features in the reference property is provided by the design of the framework.
2. Measurability: By appropriate setting of the rendering parameters, it is possible to measure the values of the dependent property at any point in the reference property: If volume rendering is used for the second property, it is sufficient to classify the dependent property as opaque at the position of interest in the reference property and as transparent at all other places.
3. Exploration and no need for segmentation: By using volume rendering, there is no a-priori need for segmenting the data sets. This enables the user to explore data sets with which he is unfamiliar. By providing facilities for the user to interactively change the classification of materials in standard volume rendering techniques, regions of interest can easily be highlighted and other parts can be faded out. However, if readily segmented data sets are available, these can be used directly.
4. Different size and resolutions of the data sets: The framework allows application of differently sized data sets, as long as no data set's size is larger than the reference property's. Different resolutions and even different coordinate systems for the different data sets cause no problems as long as there is a mapping that allows the use of the depth map generated using the reference data set together with the other data sets.
5. Relations between properties: Throughout the above discussion, the main focus was on simply locating a feature. Another very important aspect is relations between properties: For simply localizing a feature, it might be enough to add a coordinate system to the visualization. But for recognizing two properties in relation to one another it is crucial to visualize them jointly. This feature is automatically achieved with the algorithm: As both properties are shown in the same projection image, all local relations are immediately visible.
6. 3D-impression: The 3D-impression is as good as the respective rendering algorithm used for the properties.
7. Interactivity: Interactivity is achieved by the implementation as described. Furthermore, the framework is very well suited for distributed rendering [5], which allows for interactive implementations even for high quality rendering algorithms.

Although developed with direct volume rendering in mind, the framework can be used with many kinds of rendering techniques. It is possible to render the reference property and create the depth map by direct volume rendering, and to render a second property by surface rendering or a splatting technique, as long as the other technique can take advantage of the depth map.

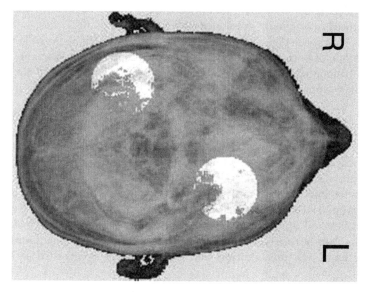

(a) From the bottom.

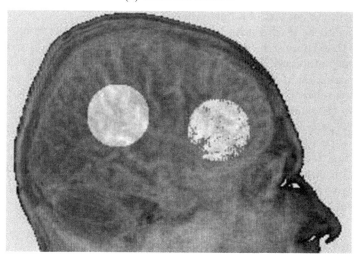

(b) From the right side.

Fig. 3. Two example renderings of a human brain (with parts of the skull re-moved) and an artificial second property (regions of suspected tumor localisa-tions). From image (a) it is perceivable that the frontal sphere from the second property is farther to the left side of the skull than the dorsal one. This is also perceivable from image (b): The frontal sphere is more fuzzy than the dorsal one because it is occluded by more tissue than the dorsal sphere. (MRI data set of the head courtesy of, and copyright by, Mark Bentum)

An implementation of this framework using the fast shear-warp volume rendering algorithm originally developed by [6] is presented in [7].

By appropriate settings of the rendering parameters, it is possible to mimic the behaviour of both the surface mapping and the transfer function approach with this framework. By defining cutting planes, even images like those of the image gallery approach can be produced.

6   Discussion

The proposed framework represents a novel apporach to the visualization of multiple properties of an object.

The most important innovation is that it is a generic approach: Arbitrary kinds of properties can be visualized, therefore the framework is not restricted to certain fields of application. This flexibility is achieved by two instruments: The mechanism of reference and dependent property on the one hand and, on the other hand, the precondition that each property is regarded as an entire volume.

Moreover, the framework supports the visualization of properties that are difficult to mentally reconstruct (like e.g. heat distributions) by visualizing such properties in the context of a reference property.

In order to be used sensibly, it is neccessary that the user is an expert in the sense that he must have an a priori knowledge of the general structure of the reference property: If the user has no knowledge of the constitution of the reference structure, it is useless to express features of the dependent property in terms of the reference property. In the medical context, this means that the user must know the anatomy of the part of the body he is examining. Furthermore, to diagnose pathologies, he must know what values of the dependent properties are to be expected at a given point in the reference structure.

After first tests, the framework appears to be a promising approach for the visualization of multiple properties of an object. We will test this framework thoroughly to improve it and to find appropiate dependent rendering techniques for different visualization purposes.

7   Conclusion

A framework for visualizing two or more properties of an object in one projection has been introduced. It allows the visualization of arbitrary combinations of properties of an object. Since the results from the first implementation were encouraging, the authors consider the dependent rendering approach to be worth further research.

References

1. Ulf Tiede, Thomas Schiemann, and Karl Heinz Höhne, "High quality rendering of attributed volume data", in *Proceedings of IEEE Visualization '98*, David Ebert, Hans Hagen, and Holly Rushmeier (eds.), IEEE Computer Society, 1998, pp. 255–262.
2. C. Rocha, J.-L. Dillenseger, and J.-L. Coatrieux, "Multi-array EEG signals mapped with three-dimensional images for clinical epilepsy studies", in *Proceedings of the 4th International Conference on Visualization in Biomedical Computing 1996*, Karl Heinz Höhne and Ron Kikinis (eds.), 1996, No. 1131 in Lecture Notes in Computer Science, pp. 467–476, Springer.
3. A. König, H. Doleisch, and E. Gröller, "Multiple views and magic mirrors - fMRI visualization of the human brain", in *Proceedings of Spring Conference on Computer Graphics and its Applications 1999 (SCCG'99)*, 1999, pp. 130–139.
4. Marc Levoy, "Efficient ray tracing of volume data", *ACM Transactions on Graphics*, vol. 9(3), pp. 245–261, July 1990.
5. Steffen Märkle and Axel Spikermann, "Distributed visualization. How to improve the quality of medical volume rendering at almost no cost", in *Proceedings of EuroPACS'98*, Joaquim Piqueras and Juan-Carlos Carreño (eds.), EuroPACS-Society, October 1998, pp. 225–228.
6. Philippe Lacroute and Marc Levoy, "Fast volume rendering using a shear-warp factorization of the viewing transformation", *Computer Graphics*, vol. 28(4), pp. 451–458, August 1994.
7. Sebastian Löbbert and Steffen Märkle, "An extension of the shear-warp volume rendering algorithm for the visualization of multiple properties of an object", to be published in *Proceedings of the 2nd IASTED International Conference on Visualization, Imaging and Image Processing (VIIP) 2002*, September 2002.

Automatic Detection of Microaneurysms in Color Fundus Images of the Human Retina by Means of the Bounding Box Closing

Thomas Walter and Jean-Claude Klein

Centre de Morphologie Mathématique
Ecole nationale supérieure des Mines de Paris
35 rue St.Honoré, 77305 Fontainebleau CEDEX, France
walter@cmm.ensmp.fr, klein@cmm.ensmp.fr,
http://cmm.ensmp.fr/~walter/

Abstract. In this paper we propose a new algorithm for the detection of microaneurysms in color fundus images of the human retina. Microaneurysms are the first unequivocal indication of Diabetic Retinopathy (DR), a severe and wide-spread eye disease. Their automatic detection may play a major role in computer assisted diagnosis of DR. We propose an algorithm that can be divided into four steps. The first step is an image enhancement technique that comprises normalization and noise reduction. The second step ist the extraction of small details that fulfill a certain criterion: This leads to the definition of the bounding box closing. Then, an automatic threshold depending on image quality is calculated. In the last step false positives are eliminated.

1 Introduction

Diabetic Retinopathy is a very severe and wide-spread eye-disease. In fact, it is the principal cause of legal blindness for the working age population of western countries. Microaneurysms are the first ophthalmoscopic sign of this disease [1]. Over and above that, their number is an indication of the progression of the disease. Their detection is therefore crucial for the diagnosis of Diabetic Retinopathy.

Because Diabetic Retinopathy becomes symptomatic only in its later stage, diabetic patients may not be aware of having been affected by the disease in its beginning. Therefore, regular retinal examinations of the risk groups are highly recommended. The costs of these examinations and the shortage of specialists, especially in rural areas, are the drawbacks of this procedure. A computer assisted approach could help to overcome these problems, because examination time and the number of specialists necessary to perform the examinations are diminished.

Furthermore, in order to monitor the disease, comparison between images taken at different examinations is necessary. Up to now, the number of microaneurysms is compared, but it would lead to a more sophisticated diagnosis, if one

A. Colosimo et al. (Eds.): ISMDA 2002, LNCS 2526, pp. 210–220, 2002.

could compare the evolution of each single lesion. Because this task can hardly be fulfilled manually, a computer assisted approach is required - consisting in detecting microaneurysms and registration of retinal images [2].

For these reasons, we think that relying on a robust and fast algorithm for the detection of microaneurysms is the crucial point of any computer assistance for the diagnosis of Diabetic Retinopathy.

2   Strategies for the Detection of Microaneurysms

2.1   Properties of Microaneurysms

Microaneurysms are tiny dilations of the capillaries (see figure 1(a)). They appear as small reddish isolated patterns of circular shape in color fundus images of the human retina [1] (see also figure 1(b)). Their diameter lies normally between $10\mu m$ and $100\mu m$, but it is always smaller than $125\mu m$. As they come from capillaries, and as capillaries are not visible in color fundus images, they appear as isolated patterns, i.e. disconnected from the vascular tree.

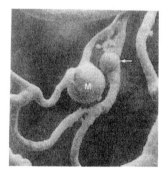
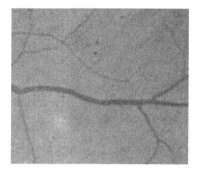

(a) A photography of microaneurysms

(b) Microaneurysms in the green channel of color fundus images.

Fig. 1. Microaneurysms in the human retina and their appearance in the green channel of color fundus images

2.2   The State of the Art

The detection of microaneurysms in fluorescein angiograms has been the subject of many publications. Detecting microaneurysms in color images is a quite similar task, even if microaneurysms appear much less contrasted than in angiograms. Unlike in color images, blood containing elements appear as bright patterns in angiograms and they are well-contrasted.

All the presented approaches can be divided into a preprocessing step (noise reduction, shade correction, image normalization, contrast enhancement), the detection of small details (potential microaneurysms, or "candidates"), a threshold and an a posteriori elimination of false positives (see figure 2).

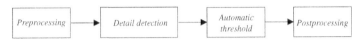

Fig. 2. The strategy for the detection of microaneurysms

In [3], the top-hat transformation $f - \gamma^{sup} f$ (with γ^{sup} the supremum of morphological openings with linear structuring elements B_i) is introduced in order to detect small peaks and to distinguish them from vessel like patterns. An a posteriori decision is based on the shape of the extracted details and their locus. In [4] and [5], a prefiltering step is added to this method (image enhancement and Gaussian filtering). Various shape properties are used to distinguish between real microaneurysms and false positives. In [6], different classification methods are compared in order to optimize the post-processing step.

3   A New Approach Based on the Bounding Box Closing

In this section we propose a new algorithm which is also based on the strategy shown in figure 2. We propose an enhancement method which comprises contrast enhancement and shade correction in one step, the bounding box closing for the detection of dark details in a gray level image, as well as a threshold technique that takes into consideration the image quality. The elimination of false positives is based on methods proposed in [3], [4].

We work on the green channel f_g of the color image, because the blood containing elements are most contrasted in this channel, as shown in [7].

3.1   Pre-processing

One of the main differences between angiographies and the green channel of color images is the lower contrast of the latter ones. Thus, enhancement techniques have to be applied. As these images are often very noisy, a compromise has to be made between contrast enhancement and noise reduction. We apply first a grey level transformation in order to enhance the contrast and then in a second step a Gaussian filter.

Let $f : D_f \subset \mathbb{Z} \to T = \{t_{min}, ..., t_{max}\}$ be a grey level image, and let $g : D_f \to U = \{u_{min}, ..., u_{max}\}$ be the enhanced image. The local contrast enhancement operator is a mapping Γ from T to U with:

$$u = \Gamma(t) = \begin{cases} a_1 \cdot t^r + b_1 & \text{,if } t \leq \mu_f(x) \\ a_2 \cdot t^r + b_2 & \text{,if } t > \mu_f(x) \end{cases}$$

with $a_1 = \frac{1}{2}\frac{u_{max}-u_{min}}{\mu_f^r - t_{min}^r}$, $b_1 = u_{min} - a_1 \cdot t_{min}^r$, $a_2 = \frac{1}{2}\frac{u_{max}-u_{min}}{t_{max}^r - \mu_f^r}$, $b_2 = u_{max} - a_2 \cdot t_{max}^r$ and $\mu_f(x)$ the mean value of f in a window $W(x)$ centered in x containing N points $\mu_f(x) = \frac{1}{N}\sum_{\xi \in W(x)} f(\xi)$.

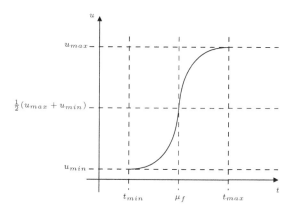

Fig. 3. The graph for the local contrast enhancement operator $\Gamma : T \to U$

The graph of this transformation is shown in figure 3. For $r = 1$ it is a linear contrast stretching and for $r \to \infty$ a local threshold operation at the mean grey level μ_f.

Applying this operator to the pixels contained in a window W has two effects: As the grey level value $g(x)$ of the enhanced image at a point x only depends on the difference between the original grey level value $f(x)$ and the mean grey level value $\mu_f(x)$ within the window W centered in x, the influence of slow grey level variations is eliminated (shade correction). Secondly, the contrast of small dark elements is enhanced even if they are situated in a dark region. If we applied the transformation shown in 3 globally, the contrast for dark elements within dark regions would be attenuated as $\frac{\partial u}{\partial t} < 1$.

The result of the proposed enhancement technique is shown in figure 4.

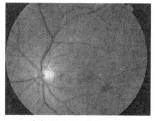

(a) Original image

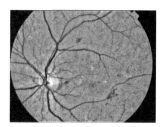

(b) Enhanced image

Fig. 4. Result of the local contrast enhancement operator (for $r = 5$)

In order to attenuate the noise, but to preserve the microaneursyms, we filter the image with a gaussian. This method has been discussed in [8]; the gaussian filter can be seen as a matched filter, because the shape of the microaneurysms can be modeled as a two dimensional gaussian. Hence, we obtain the preprocessed image p by convolving the enhanced image g with a Gaussian convolution kernel G: $p = G * g$.

3.2   Detection of Holes - The Bounding Box Closing

As stated in 2.1, microaneurysms appear as isolated circular patterns of a diameter smaller than λ, and they appear darker than the background.

In Mathematical Morphology we interpret grey level images as topographic surfaces and hence, dark details correspond to holes (or valleys). Hence, in terms of Mathematical Morphology, microaneurysms can be modeled as "holes" of a diameter smaller than λ. The problem is now to conceive a transformation that is able to extract these details.

A common method to extract dark details in an image is the Morphological top-hat transform $\phi f - f$ in which ϕf is an algebraic closing, i.e. an increasing, idempotent and extensive transformation, that is conceived in such a way that dark details that fulfill the criterion are removed.

Different approaches have been presented for such a closing, but they have some imperfections: The morphological closing eliminates small vessels (ditches) as well, the infimum of morphological closings with linear structuring elements does better, but it removes also tortuous patterns from the image.

Therefore, we propose a new closing ϕ_λ° which eliminates all holes in an image with a diameter smaller than λ. In a first step, we define a binary closing that "fills all holes" in a binary image for which the criterion holds, and then we extend this binary operator to grey level images applying it successively on every threshold of the image.

The Diameter of a Connected Set: We define the maximal diameter of a connected set $X \subset \mathbb{Z}^2$:

Definition 1. *Let $X \subset \mathbb{Z}^2$ be a connected set, x and y two points and $d(x,y)$ the distance between them. We define the maximal diameter of X as:*

$$\alpha(X) = \bigvee_{x,y \in X} d(x,y)$$

In the following, we refer to the block distance: If $x = (x_1, x_2), y = (y_1, y_2) \in \mathbb{Z}^2$ points and x_1, x_2 and y_1, y_2 their coordinates respectively, the block distance can be written as $d(x,y) = |x_1 - y_1| \vee |x_2 - y_2|$. Hence, the maximal diameter defined in definition 1 is, for this distance, the size of the "bounding box" into which the set X fits.

The Bounding Box Closing for Binary Images: The binary closing ϕ_λ° should eliminate all "holes" (connected components of X^c, with $(\cdot)^c$ the inversion operator) in the binary image X that have a diameter smaller than or equal to λ, or in other words, the resulting set only has holes with diameter larger than λ.

Let $C_x(A)$ be the connected component of the set A that contains x if $x \in A$ end the empty set $\emptyset$ elsewhere. Then we can define the binary bounding box closing:

Definition 2. *Let $X \subset \mathbb{Z}^2$ be a set and $(\cdot)^c$ the inversion operator. The binary bounding box closing ϕ_λ° is defined by:*

$$\phi_\lambda^\circ(X) = X \cup \{x \in X^c | \alpha\,[C_x(X^c)] \le \lambda\} \tag{1}$$

This is equivalent to $[\phi_\lambda^\circ]^c(X) = \{x \in X^c | \alpha\,[C_x(X^c)] > \lambda\}$. It can be seen easily that this operator is *increasing, idempotent* and *extensive*, and that it is therefore an algebraic closing. As it is increasing, we can extend this closing to grey level images.

The Bounding Box Closing for Grey Level Images: Let X_t^- be the set of all pixels with a grey level smaller than or equal to t: $X_t^- = \{x \in D_f | f(x) \le t\}$. Considering the image f as a topographic surface, we can interpret X_t^- as the set of pixels belonging to "lakes", after the image has been flooded up to the level t (see figure 5). Hence, $C_x(X_t^-)$ denotes the lake, to which x belongs, if x belongs to the flooded part of the image. The bounding box closing assigns to

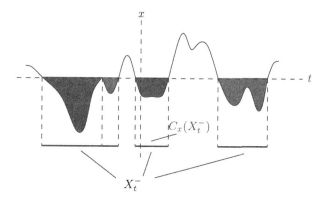

Fig. 5. Flooding of a function at level t. X_t^- corresponds to the lakes flooded up to t, $C_x(X_t^-)$ is the lake containing the point x.

each pixel the infimum of level $t \ge f(x)$, up to which the corresponding lake has to be flooded so that its diameter is greater than λ (see also figure 6).

Definition 3. *Let $f : D_f \rightarrow T$ be a grey level image. We define the bounding box closing of a grey level image:*

$$\phi_\lambda^\circ f(x) = \inf\{t \geq f(x) | \alpha \left[C_x(X_t^-) \right] > \lambda\} \qquad (2)$$

For the implementation of this algorithm, we flood the image starting with the local minima, and at each level we test for each lake $C_x(X_t^-)$, if its diameter is larger than λ. If this condition is met, the actual grey level is the stop level for this lake. If a lake meets another lake before the condition is met, the two lakes are fused and considered as one lake in the following (see figure 5). In that way we proceed until the whole image has been flooded. This approach is close to the area opening presented in [9].

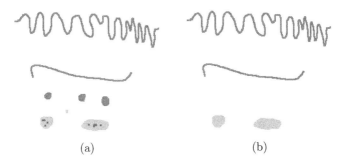

(a)   (b)

Fig. 6. An example for the bounding box closing of a grey level image. All dark details ("holes") of diameter smaller than 20 pixels are removed ("filled"). Tortuous patterns, ditches and larger holes remain unchanged.

We apply this closing on the prefiltered image p. ϕ_λ° removes just the details we are looking for. Hence, we calculate the top-hat associated to this closing $TH(p) = \phi_\lambda^\circ p - p$, and we obtain an image that contains all dark details of p with a diameter smaller than λ: Microaneurysms and other features having similar properties (noise and small hemorrhages).

3.3   The Automatic Threshold

Once the dark details detected, we have to apply a threshold in order to distinguish between real microaneurysms and noise of low amplitude. It has been stated that applying a low fix threshold constant for all images leads in many cases to a lot of false positives [4]. Applying a histogram based threshold like in [2] and [5] one detects microaneurysms even if there are none, and assessing the image quality a priori and applying a quality dependent threshold introduces subjectivity and irreproducibility [3], if the assessment is not automatic. However, image quality is hard to be determined automatically.

We have observed that all retinal images are corrupted by pixel noise. This noise is sure not to represent important features in the retina, and it is an indication of both the amount of noise and the contrast of the image. The higher the amount of noise the higher we have to choose the threshold in order not to obtain a lot of false positives, and the better the contrast of an image the higher we *can* choose the threshold without missing a lot of microaneurysms. Hence, we follow a heuristic approach: We determine the best threshold for 25 images and we compare them with the mean values of the pepper noise (for extraction of the pepper noise we make use of the technique proposed in [10]). The result is shown in figure 7.

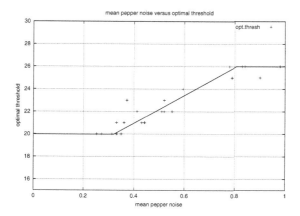

Fig. 7. The optimal thresholds versus mean pepper noise

3.4   Elimination of False Positives

Many shape characteristics have been proposed in the literature [4], [5] in order to distinguish between true microaneurysms and false positives (e.g. the perimeter, circularity etc.) in angiographies. However, we found that most of these characteristics are meaningful only for high resolution images. Over and above that, they must rely on a robust segmentation algorithm for the candidate regions, that can easily be conceived for angiographies, but not for color images because of low contrast. We found the best results for the following criteria:

- *The position*: The microaneurysms cannot be situated neither on the vascular tree nor on the optic disc. Hence, we detect the vessels and the optic disc [11] and we remove all candidates on these features.
- *The area*: Often we have a relatively high amount of high amplitude pixel noise. Hence, we simply remove all candidates that have an area smaller than a certain value (we assumed in our images, that the area of the candidates must be larger than 3 pixels).

– *The local contrast criterion* (similar to that proposed in [5]): We calculate the difference between the mean value within the candidate region and the mean value on the outside of it. If this criterion is smaller than a parameter κ, we reject the candidate. In our case, good results were found for $\kappa = 8$.

4   Results

At the moment we cannot present a clinical validation of the algorithm, but just a preliminary test. The algorithm has been tested on 5 images taken with a SONY color video 3CCD camera on a Topcon TRC 50 IA retinograph (resolution 640×480). The images contained 133 microaneurysms (marked by a human grader). Of these microaneurysms, 86.4% were detected by the proposed algorithm. We also detected false positives (FP), so that the predictive value, i.e. the ratio $\frac{TP}{TP+FP}$ with TP the correctly classified microaneurysms (true positives) was 74.8%[1].

Most of these false positives were situated on bigger hemorrhages or on very small low contrasted vessels that have not been detected by the vessel detection algorithm. More sensitive algorithms for detection of these features could improve the performance of the presented algorithm considerably. Microaneurysms can also easily be confounded with intraretinal microvascular abnormalities and small hemorrhages, but it might be very hard for an algorithm to distinguish between these lesions, because even for human graders, the distinction is sometimes hard to make.

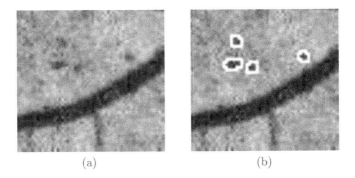

(a)   (b)

Fig. 8. An example for detected microaneurysms

Most of the missed microaneurysms were situated very close to vessels. In this case, they are connected to the vascular tree (or the hemorrhage) by the

---

[1] We could not determine the specificity because the TN (number of true negatives) cannot be determined of course. The predictive value is the probability that a detected microaneurysm is really a microaneurysm

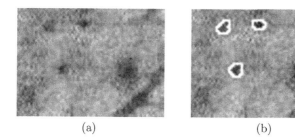

(a)   (b)

Fig. 9. An example for detected microaneurysms

prefiltering step and cannot be detected by the bounding box closing. This remains an unresolved problem that has been reported also by other authors. One way to improve the algorithm is the application of sharpening operators that are able to enhance the separation between vessel and microaneurysm.

Compared to results found in [8] and [4][2], we obtain a slightly better sensitivity (the authors obtain 82%) , but the difference is not significant as we have not tested the algorithm on a large image data base yet. Over and above that, there is a trade-off between sensitivity and the number of false positives in such a way that a greater sensitivity can be achieved by a higher number of false positives. Indeed, in [4] the authors obtain 5.7 false positives per image, we obtain 7.7 with the proposed method.

Figures 8 and 9 show examples for the results obtained by the presented algorithm (the images are enhanced for better visibility). In figure 9, the detected microaneurysm on the bottom right corner may be a small hemorrhage. However, even for human graders, the difference is hardly visible.

5   Conclusion and Perspectives

A new algorithm for the detection of microaneurysms has been presented comprising image enhancement, the bounding box closing for detail extraction, an automatic threshold and a postfiltering step. The performance is satisfying, but the clinical validation is still in progress.

However, the algorithm could be improved using more accurate algorithms for detection of vessels and hemorrhages. A second way to improve the performance of the algorithm is the optimization of the last step: More properties could be used, and sophisticated classification methods comprising a learning phase could be applied.

This algorithm shall be a part of a bigger software tool which is under development. It shall comprise detection of other pathologies related to DR, detection of the main features in the human eye, image registration and an automatic evaluation of the evolution of the single lesions.

---

[2] The authors work on angiograms, not on color images.

References

[1] P. Massin, A. Erginay, and A. Gaudric, *Rétinopathie Diabéthique*, vol. 1, Paris, elsevier edition, 2000.

[2] F. Zana, *Une approche morphologique pour les détections et Bayesienne pour le recalage d'images multimodales: Application aux images rétiniennes*, thesis, ENSMP, CMM, May 1999.

[3] B. Lay, *Analyse automatique des images angiofluorographiques au cours de la rétinopathie diabétique*, thesis, ENSMP, CMM, June 1983.

[4] T. Spencer et al., "An image processing strategy for the segmentation and quantification of mycroaneurysms in fluorescein angiograms of the ocular fundus," *Computers and biomedical research*, vol. 29, pp. 284–302, 1996.

[5] A. M. Mendonça et al., "Automatic segmentation of microaneurysms in retinal angiograms of diabetic patients," *Proc. ICIAP 99*, pp. 728–733, 1999.

[6] A. Frame et al., "A comparison of computer based classification methods applied to the detection of microaneurysms in ophthalmic fluorescein angiograms," *Computers in Biology and Medecine*, vol. 28, pp. 225–238, 1998.

[7] T. Hellstedt, E. Vesti, and I. Immonen, "Identification of individual microaneurysms: A comparison between fluorescein angiograms and red-free and colour photographs," *Graefe's Arch Clin Exp Ophtalmol*, vol. 234, pp. 13–17, 1996.

[8] M. J. Cree, J. A. Olson, K. C. McHardy, J. V. Forrester, and P. F. Sharp, "Automated microaneurysm detection," *International Conference on Image Processing (ICIP)*, sep 1996.

[9] L. Vincent, "Morphological area openings and closings for grayscale images," *Shape in picture, NATO workshop, Driebergen*, Sep 1992.

[10] P. Soille, *Morphological Image Analysis*, Springer-Verlag, 1999.

[11] T. Walter and J.-C. Klein, "Segmentation of color fundus images of the human retina: Detection of the optic disc and the vascular tree using morphological techniques," *proc. of ISMDA 2001*, pp. 282–287, Oct 2001.

Author Index

Lecture Notes in Computer Science

For information about Vols. 1–2425
please contact your bookseller or Springer-Verlag